5 Explosive SECRETS
that Guarantee Good HEALTH

Published by Sebastijan Prislan at CreateSpace.



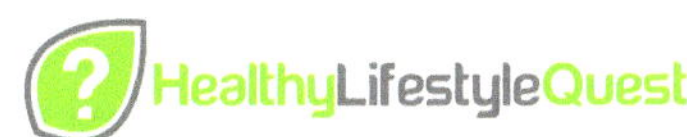


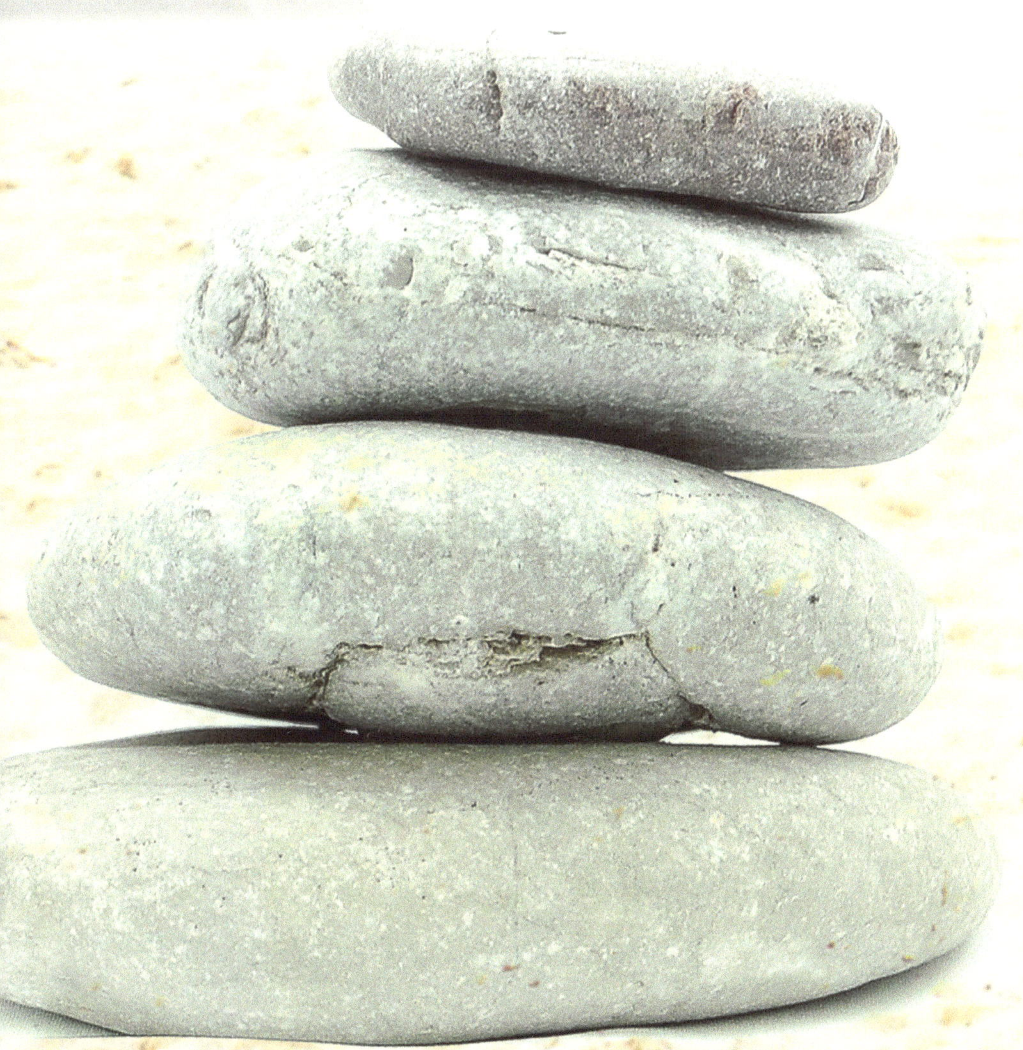

# 5 Explosive SECRETS that Guarantee Good HEALTH

## Legal & Disclaimer

The information contained in this book is not designed to replace or take the place of any form of medicine or professional medical advice. The information in this book has been provided for educational and entertainment purposes only.

The information contained in this book has been compiled from sources deemed reliable, and it is accurate to the best of the Author's knowledge; however, the Author cannot guarantee its accuracy and validity and cannot be held liable for any errors or omissions. Changes are periodically made to this book. You must consult your doctor or get professional medical advice before using any of the suggested remedies, techniques, or information in this book.

Upon using the information contained in this book, you agree to hold harmless the Author from and against any damages, costs, and expenses, including any legal fees potentially resulting from the application of any of the information provided by this guide. This disclaimer applies to any damages or injury caused by the use and application, whether directly or indirectly, of any advice or information presented, whether for breach of contract, tort, negligence, personal injury, criminal intent, or under any other cause of action.

You agree to accept all risks of using the information presented inside this book. You need to consult a professional medical practitioner in order to ensure you are both able and healthy enough to participate in this program.

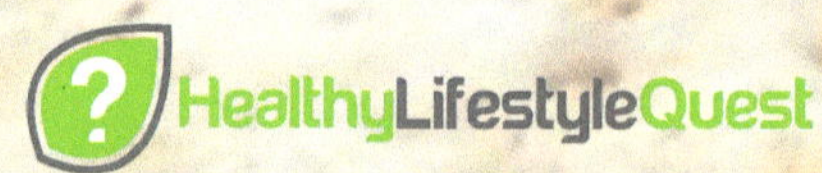

# Contents



**+ Bonus Pages**

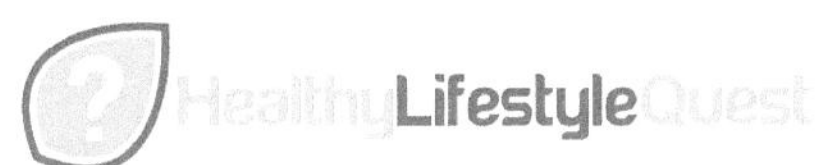

# Welcome!

Get ready to delve into the secrets of health and experience a new level in physical and emotional health.

Everyone desires good health yet most people are not ready to pay the price required to get it.  Another category of people is ready to pay the price yet lack the information with which to act.

By reading this book, you are in the latter category.

This book has been written with you in mind.

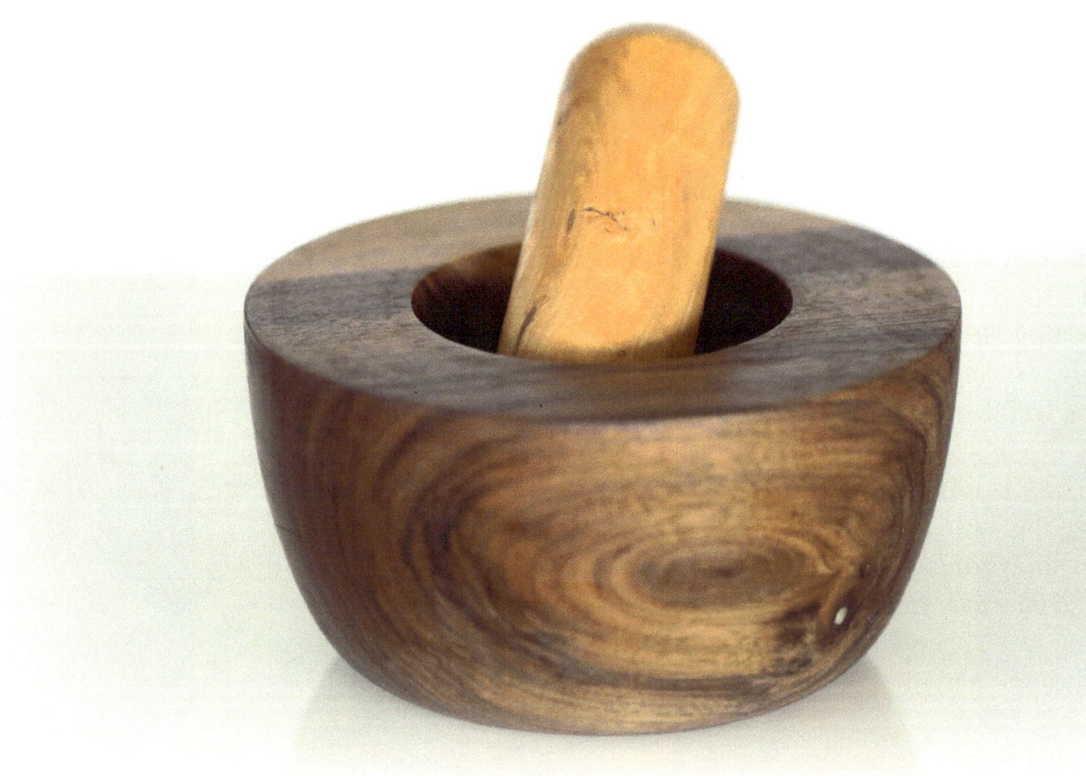

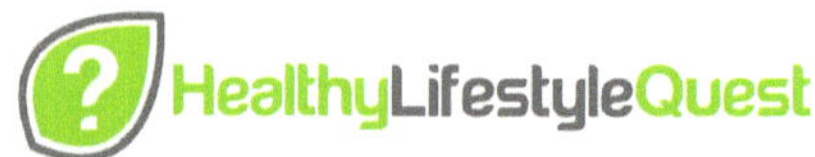

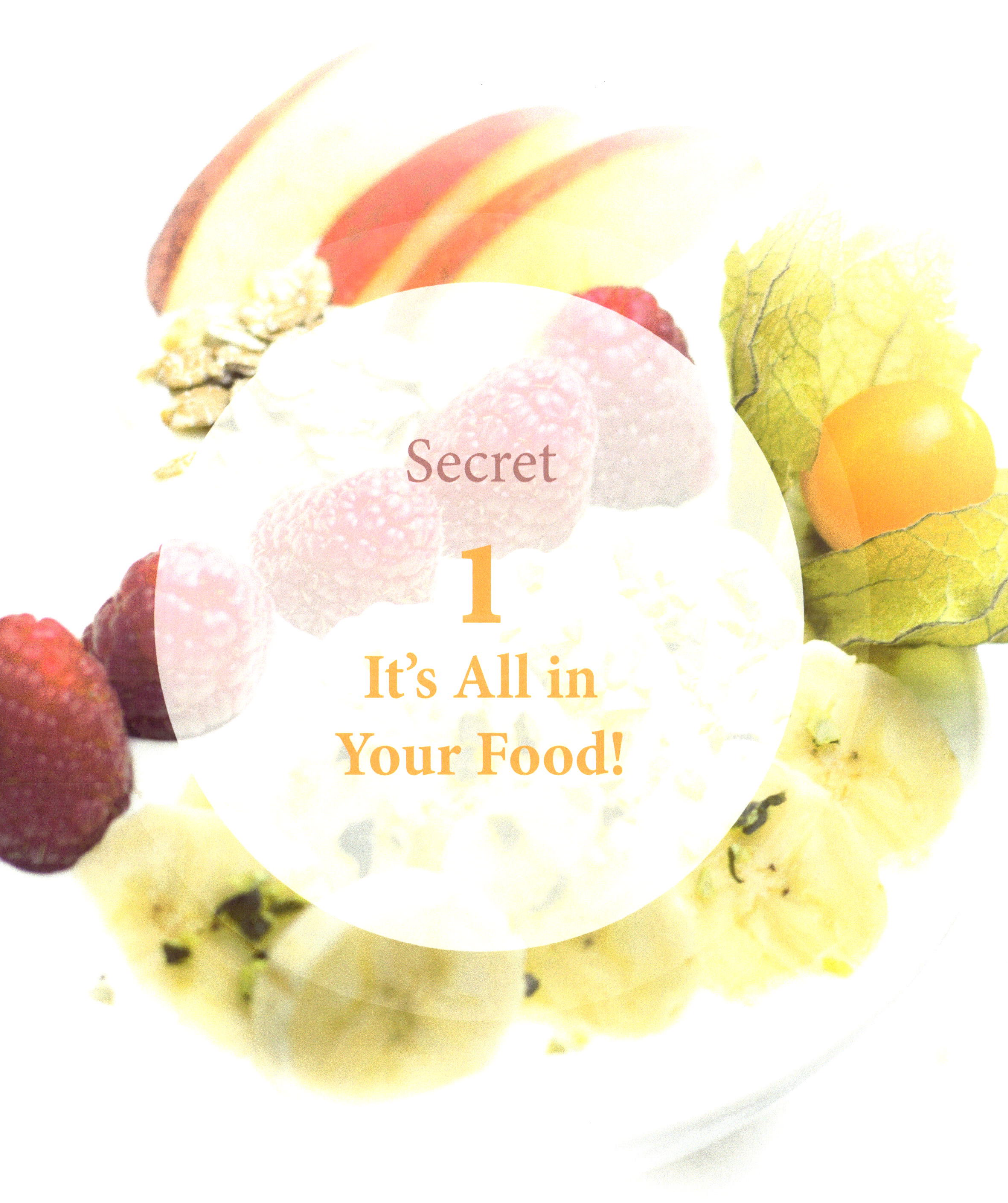

Secret

1

It's All in
Your Food!

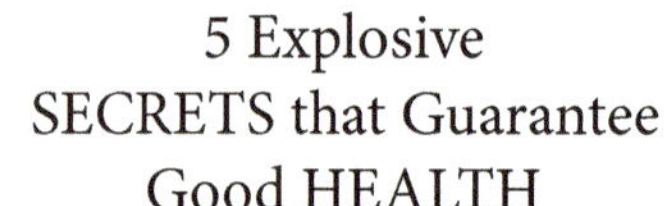

# Diet, Food and Life Expectancy

**What's diet got to do with it?** Actually, a whole lot. There is an intricate web linking your diet, type of food you eat with your life expectancy. All seem to be part of the package. Startling statistics from the World Health Organization indicate that diabetes, cardiovascular disease, cancer, obesity, osteoporosis, and dental disease are major diet-related diseases. The causes of these diseases is rooted in unhealthy diets and lifestyles.

**Healthy food choices typically result in the body feeling light and good while tiredness and sluggish feeling result from consumption of sugary and heavy foods.**

If we know this, why then do these diseases persist? Perhaps we don't really have all the information we need. For instance, many people do not realise that **the average life expectancy is approximately 26, 950 days.**

**Now, what if you are able to extend this time and live longer?** You ask how. Well, it is as simple as eating right using the proper diet. Okay, if this still sounds a little bit fuzzy to you, let's bring it down to earth a little. According to a National Geographic study, a common denominator was found in the life expectancies of three distinctly different societies. The first society was in the Russian mountains while the other two, Okinawa, Loma Linda in Japan and California respectively.

**This common denominator was their diet which was predominantly plant-based.** Of course, other studies have indicated over time that **people who adopt a plant-based diet tend to increase life expectancy by almost eight years.**

You are probably wondering if you can get good food out there. Most that float around the TV ads are just the same old fat and sodium-saturated, over-processed foods that pump you full of calories without adding a whit of nutrients. The fact is, there are over 100,000 healthy foods available to you but then, you need to have the proper knowledge of them and how to use them optimally.

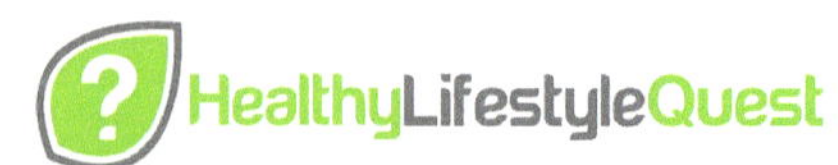

# The Right Diet

**Is there really a 'right diet'?**

Yes, there right diets out there for you. Having established the existence of right diets (proper diets that suit you), it stands to reason that the opposite also exists.

Our focus however, is on the right one.

The right diet thus incorporates the right amounts of carbs, proteins, fat and diverse nutrients required for your body to work optimally.

Still wondering what diets would work for you?

Here are a few to choose from...

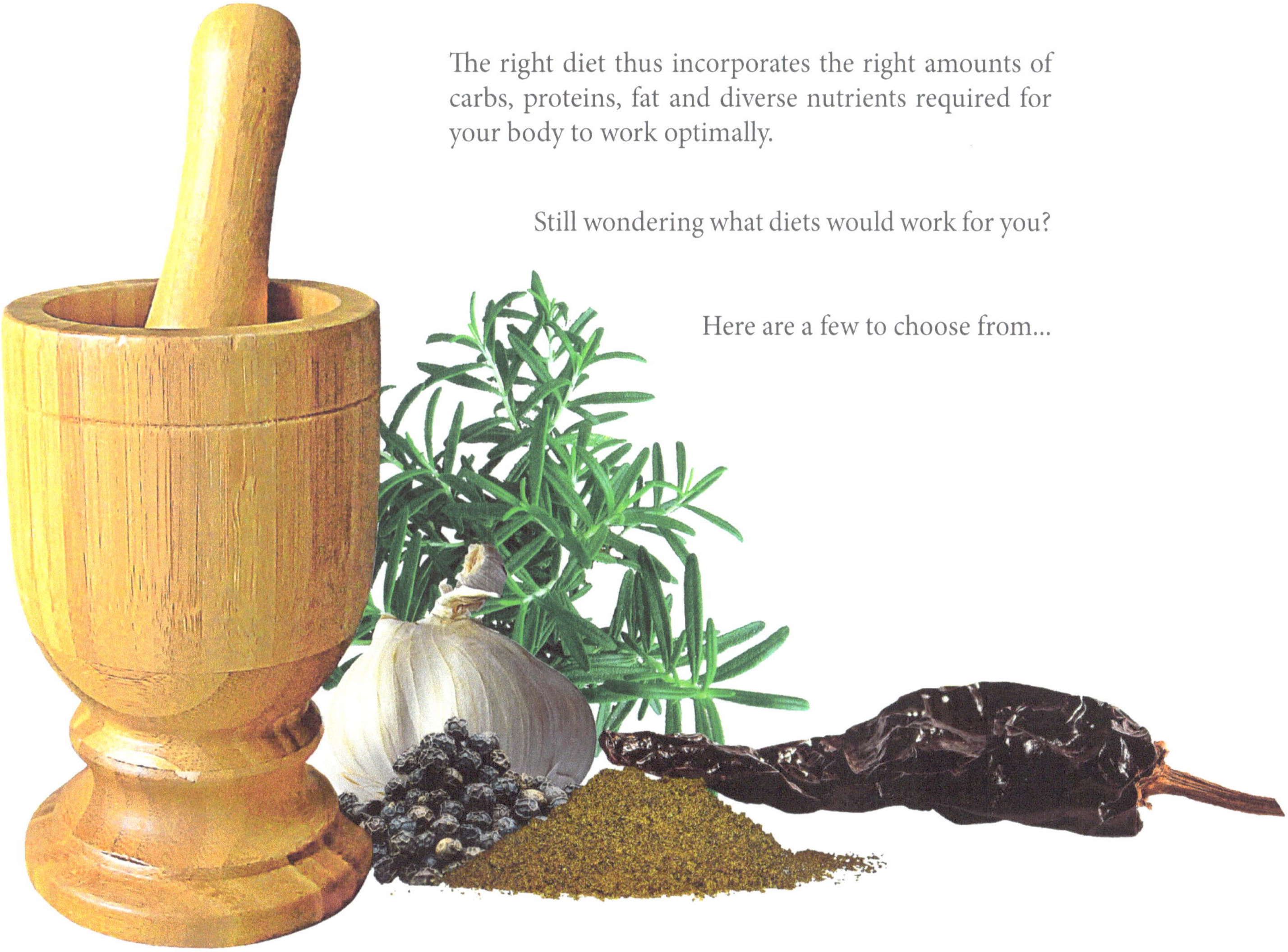

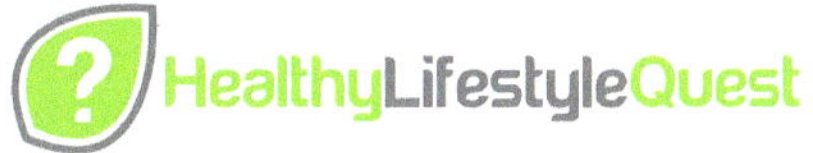

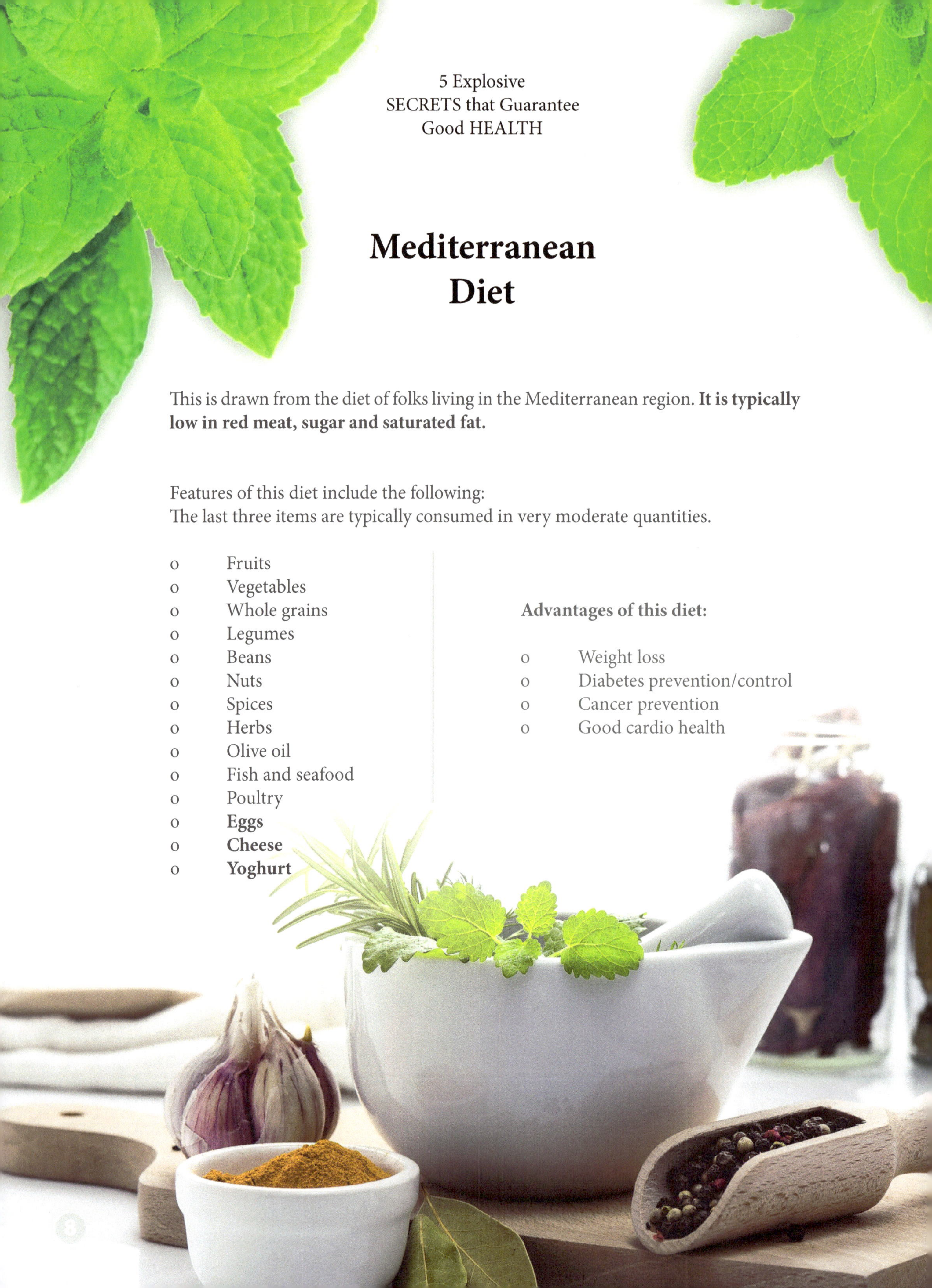



# Mediterranean Diet

This is drawn from the diet of folks living in the Mediterranean region. **It is typically low in red meat, sugar and saturated fat.**

Features of this diet include the following:
The last three items are typically consumed in very moderate quantities.

o  Fruits
o  Vegetables
o  Whole grains
o  Legumes
o  Beans
o  Nuts
o  Spices
o  Herbs
o  Olive oil
o  Fish and seafood
o  Poultry
o  **Eggs**
o  **Cheese**
o  **Yoghurt**

**Advantages of this diet:**

o  Weight loss
o  Diabetes prevention/control
o  Cancer prevention
o  Good cardio health

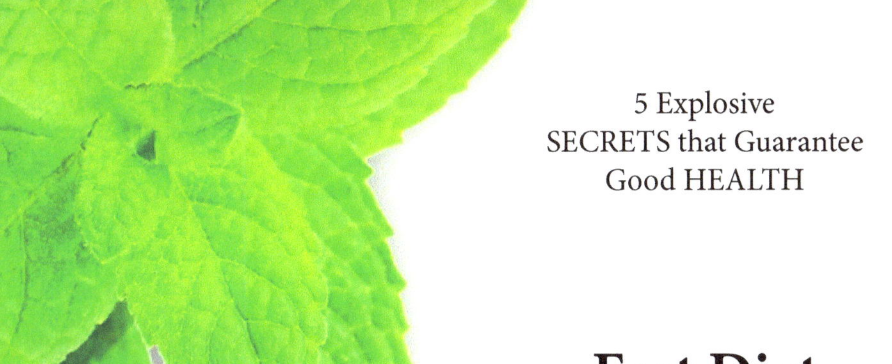



# Fast Diet

Popularized by Michael Mosley and Mimi Spencer, journalist turned doctor and journalist respectively, this diet has garnered quite a decent following.

**It generally involves the significant slicing of calories consumed two days in a week hence its alternate name; the 5:2 (or Intermittent Fast) Diet.**

The logic behind this diet is that by adopting an intermittent fast pattern, the body is compelled to enter maintenance mode thus utilizing fat from its reserves. This leads to weight loss and optimization of body resources.

**Therefore, you can eat normally for five days a week but on two separate days of the week, you slash your calories intake to a quarter.** The recommended calories intake on the fast days are 600 and 500 for men and women respectively.

Features of this diet include:

o    Skinless chicken
o    Nuts
o    Legumes
o    Steamed white fish
o    Tofu
o    Seeds
o    Fruits
o    Vegetables
o    Eggs

**Advantages of this diet:**

o    Weight loss
o    Chronic diseases prevention

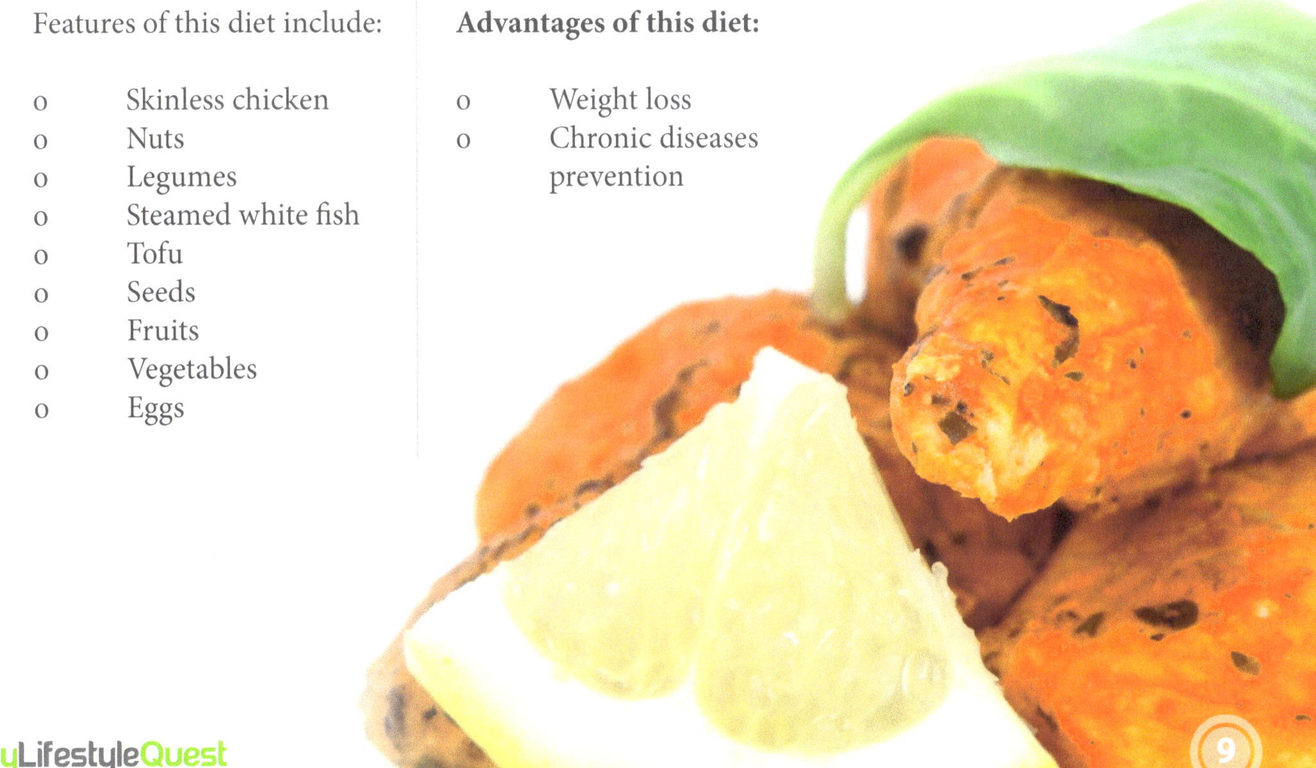

# Flexitarian Diet

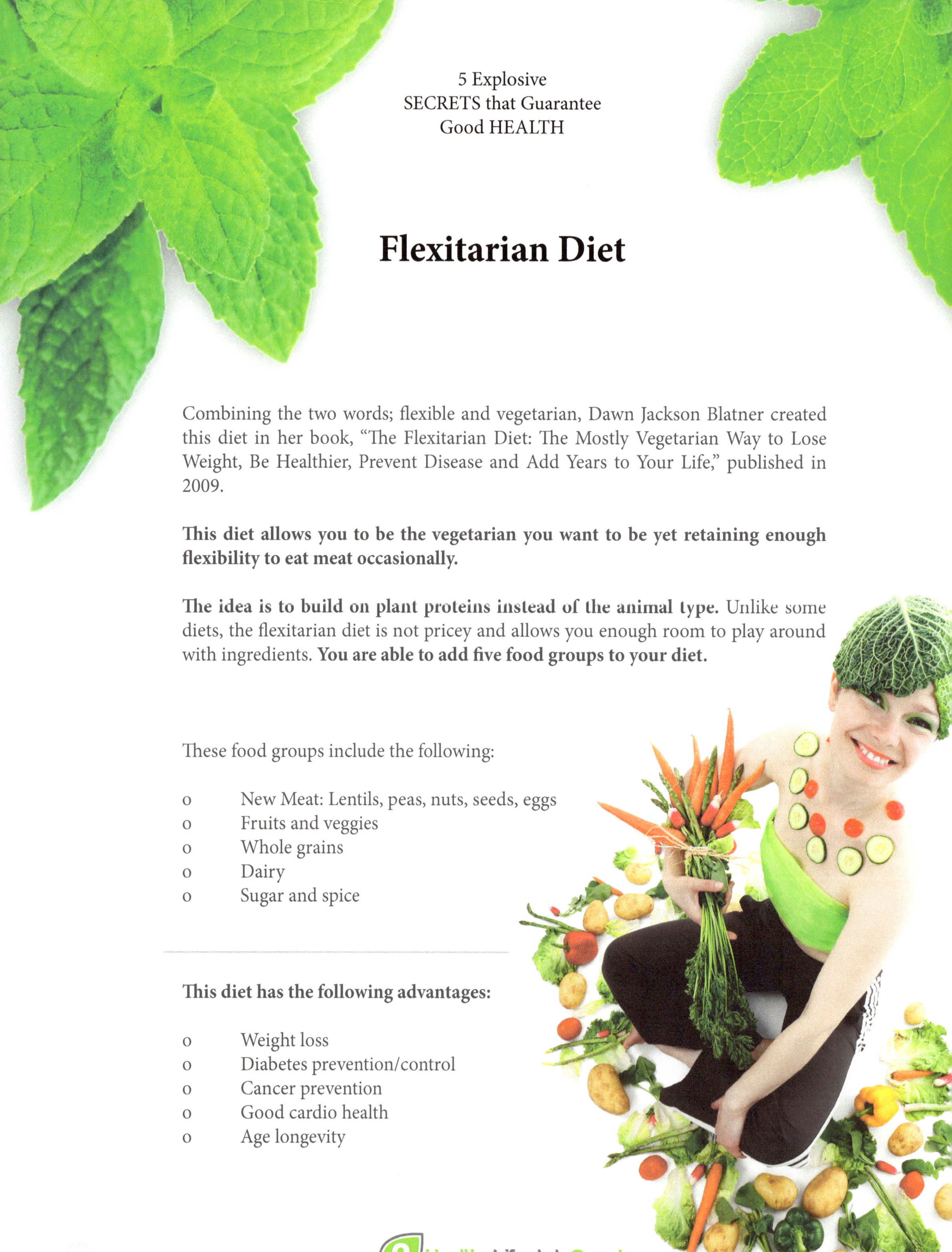

Combining the two words; flexible and vegetarian, Dawn Jackson Blatner created this diet in her book, "The Flexitarian Diet: The Mostly Vegetarian Way to Lose Weight, Be Healthier, Prevent Disease and Add Years to Your Life," published in 2009.

**This diet allows you to be the vegetarian you want to be yet retaining enough flexibility to eat meat occasionally.**

**The idea is to build on plant proteins instead of the animal type.** Unlike some diets, the flexitarian diet is not pricey and allows you enough room to play around with ingredients. **You are able to add five food groups to your diet.**

These food groups include the following:

o     New Meat: Lentils, peas, nuts, seeds, eggs
o     Fruits and veggies
o     Whole grains
o     Dairy
o     Sugar and spice

**This diet has the following advantages:**

o     Weight loss
o     Diabetes prevention/control
o     Cancer prevention
o     Good cardio health
o     Age longevity

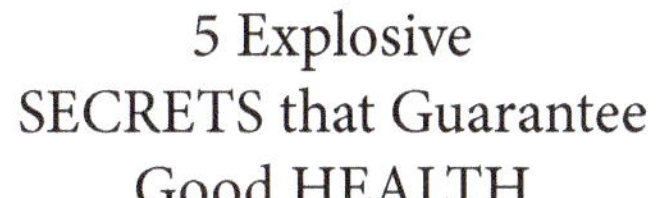

# Life-Saving Habits to Adopt Good Diet

Like most people, you are probably a creature of habit. Habits can make or mar your weight control/loss program thus <u>the key is developing the right habits.</u>

**This is one of the best kept secrets of good dieting.**

Here are some of them:

o    **Eat Plenty of Produce:** If your calories intake per day is about 2,000 calories, you should ensure you also consume 2½ cups of vegetables as well as 2 cups of fruits with it. The nutrient and fiber content of various produce such as legumes and fruits are a rich source of vital compounds needed for body growth and development.

o    **Consume More Food Instead of Supplements:** While supplements may be useful to the body, it is very important to ensure consumption of food as it contains more nutrients that are organic. These are very beneficial to the body processes.

o    **Reduce Sodium and Increase Potassium Intake:** High blood pressure easily results from excessive intake of sodium. The sodium intake for the average person should not exceed 2,300 milligrams per day. Potassium on the other hand, reduces blood pressure and can be found in foods like potatoes, yoghurt, bananas, beans and citrus fruits.

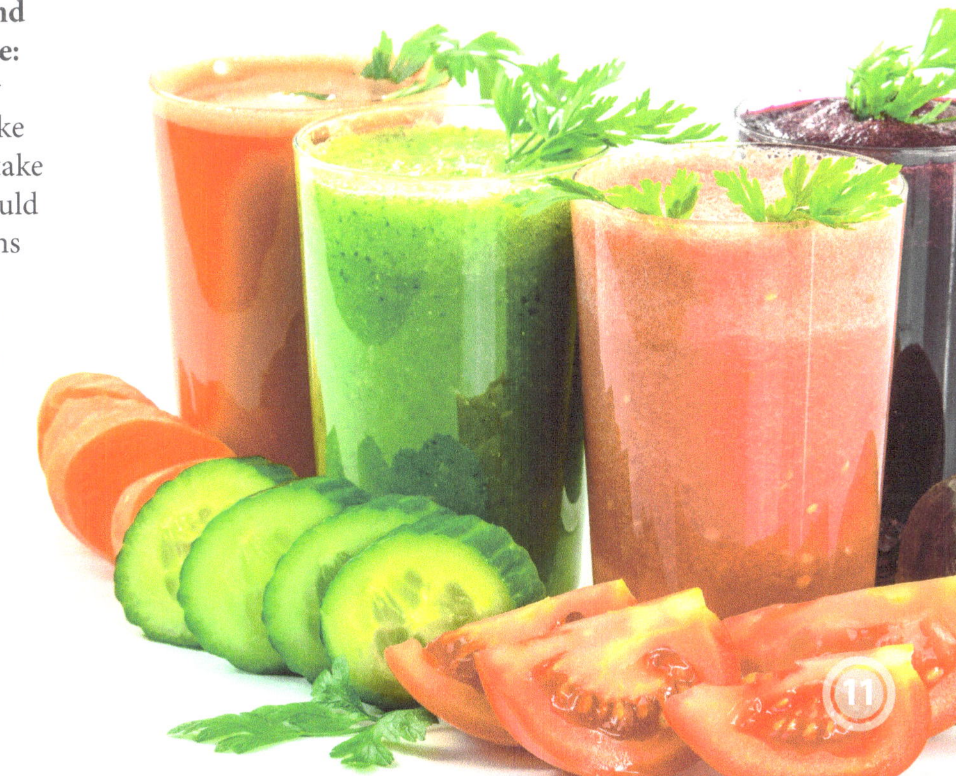

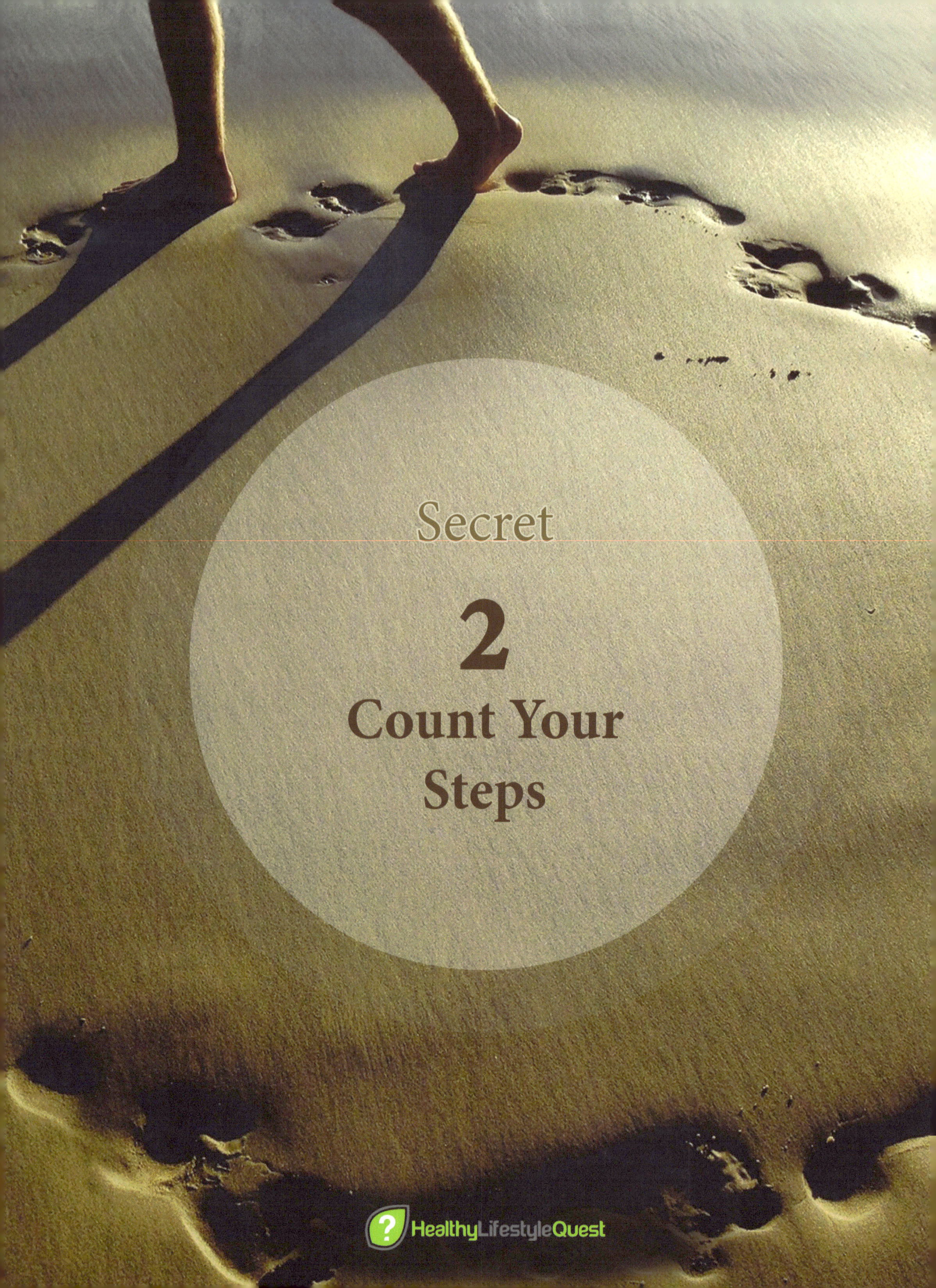

Secret

2

Count Your

Steps

HealthyLifestyleQuest

# staying on the Move...

**You may ask; should I really avoid a sedentary lifestyle? The answer is yes.**

It is vital to avoid a sedentary lifestyle and clock some distance with your feet. If you still feel the need for a kind of validation, here are a few.

**For starters, the recommendation of the UK National Obesity Forum is anything between 7,000 to 10,000 steps daily to accomplish moderate activity.**

The Japanese Ministry of Health, Labour and Welfare similarly recommends between **8,000 and 10,000 steps daily** for the same reason.

Any lingering doubts in your mind may be dispelled by the World Health Organization statistic naming **inactivity as being responsible for nine percent of premature deaths thus making it the fourth biggest killer of adults.**

Studies have continued to indicate the necessity of frequent movement such as walking to the body.

**The risk of stroke in men over sixty years old has been found to reduce by simply taking daily walks.**

Furthermore, more studies are revealing the dangers of long periods of sitting to including potential cardiovascular and muscular defects.

Additionally, it has been discovered that people who sit for long periods are more susceptible to diabetes or heart disease than people who sit for less periods.

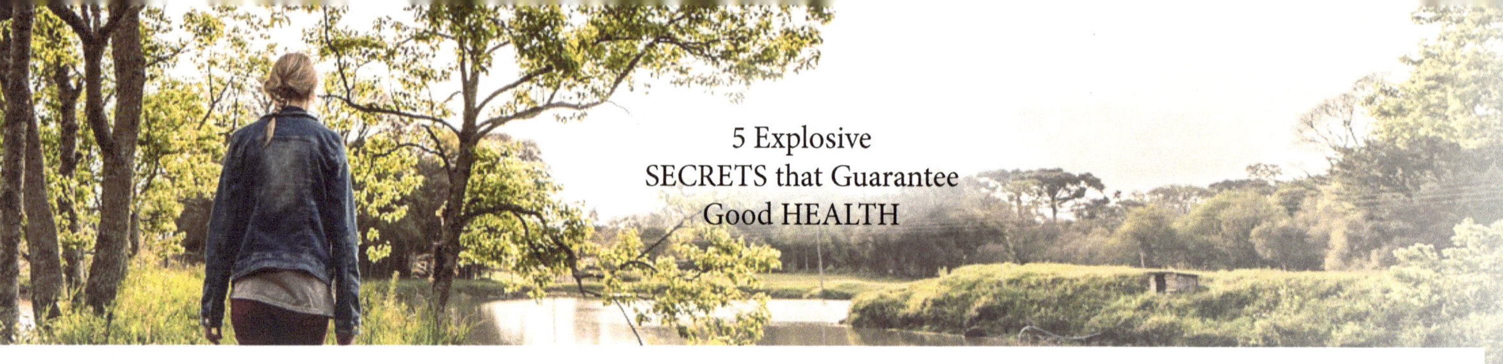


# Understanding Body Mass Index (BMI)

**This is the standard method for measurement of overweight and obesity based on the relationship between body weight and height.**

While it does not directly measure excess body fat, it provides a more accurate measurement by analyzing the weight-height relationship instead of relying solely on weight.

What is the link between BMI and inactivity?
As already mentioned above, inactivity has been found to be responsible for almost ten percent of premature deaths and overweight is largely a function of inactivity.

**BMI therefore helps to accurately determine how much fat you have as well as how much of it you have to lose.**

The risks of having a high BMI include the following:

o        High blood pressure
o        Heart disease
o        High cholesterol and blood lipids (ldl)
o        Type 2 diabetes
o        Sleep apnea
o        Osteoarthritis
o        Female infertility
o        Gastroesophageal reflux (Gerd)
o        Urinary stress incontinence

**The summary is this;**

you have got to watch your BMI and use it as a basis for determining the amount of body movement you require.

**As mentioned above, a rule of the thumb is to go with 10,000 steps per day by walking in addition to other body movement such as simple yoga.**

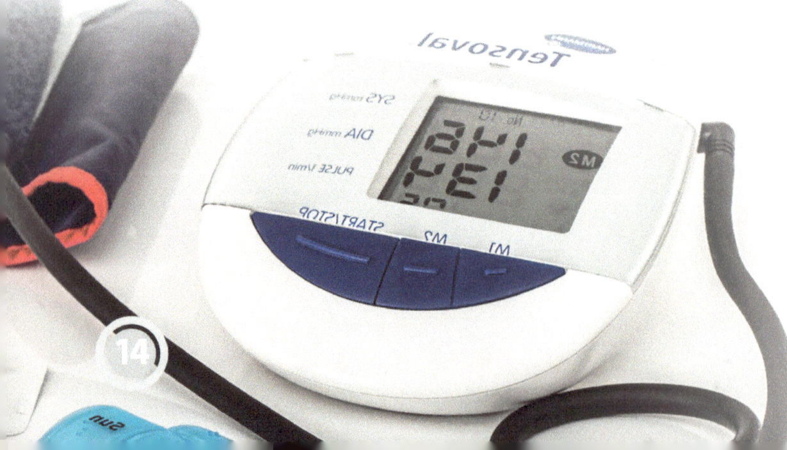



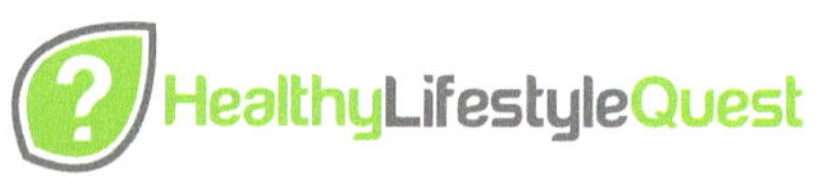

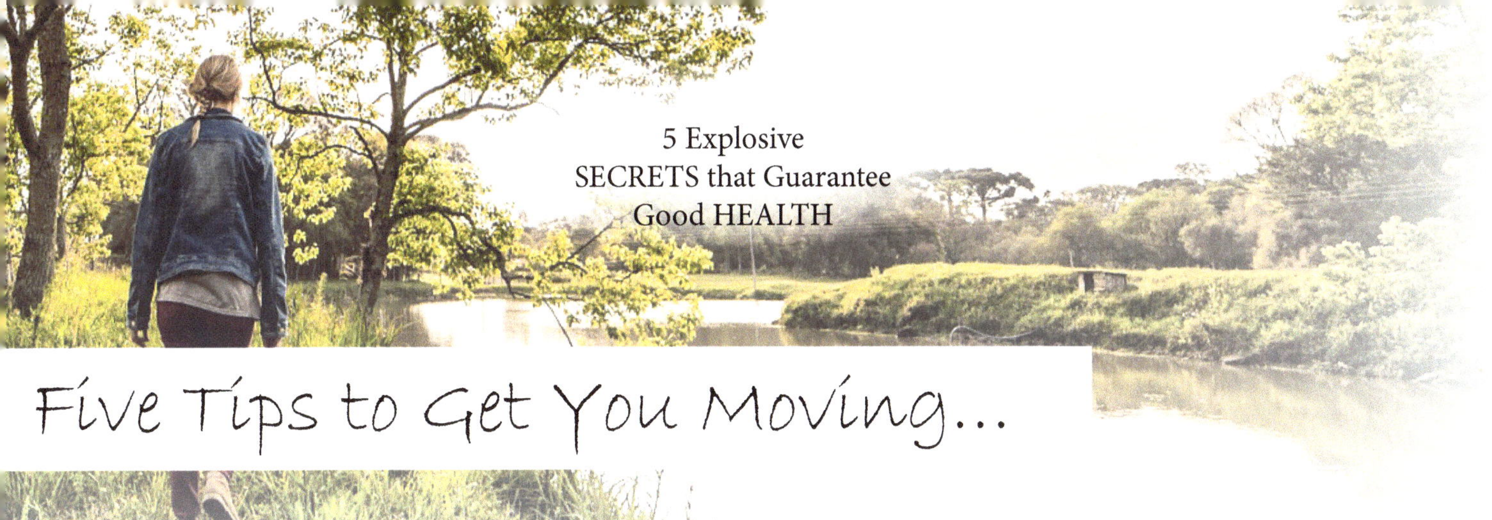


# Five Tips to Get You Moving…

As you must have gleaned from the earlier parts of this book, **you have to ensure frequent body movement in order to stay fit and healthy. This section of the book is to show you how.**

o	**Take the Stairs:** Of course, you enjoy the early morning greetings and banter with your colleagues in the elevator. However, you are better off taking the stairs for the sake of fitness. You may puff a little at the beginning but it gets better and easier once you start. Oh, you can still pop into your colleagues' offices (that's walking!) to say hi.

o	**Park Your Car Away from the Entrance:** Don't be in a hurry to grab that coveted spot close to the office entrance just to avoid the long walk from the end of the park. The fact is, the person parking over there may be gaining more than you by walking that distance. Swap lazy stroll for a walk and fitness. It's sure worth it!

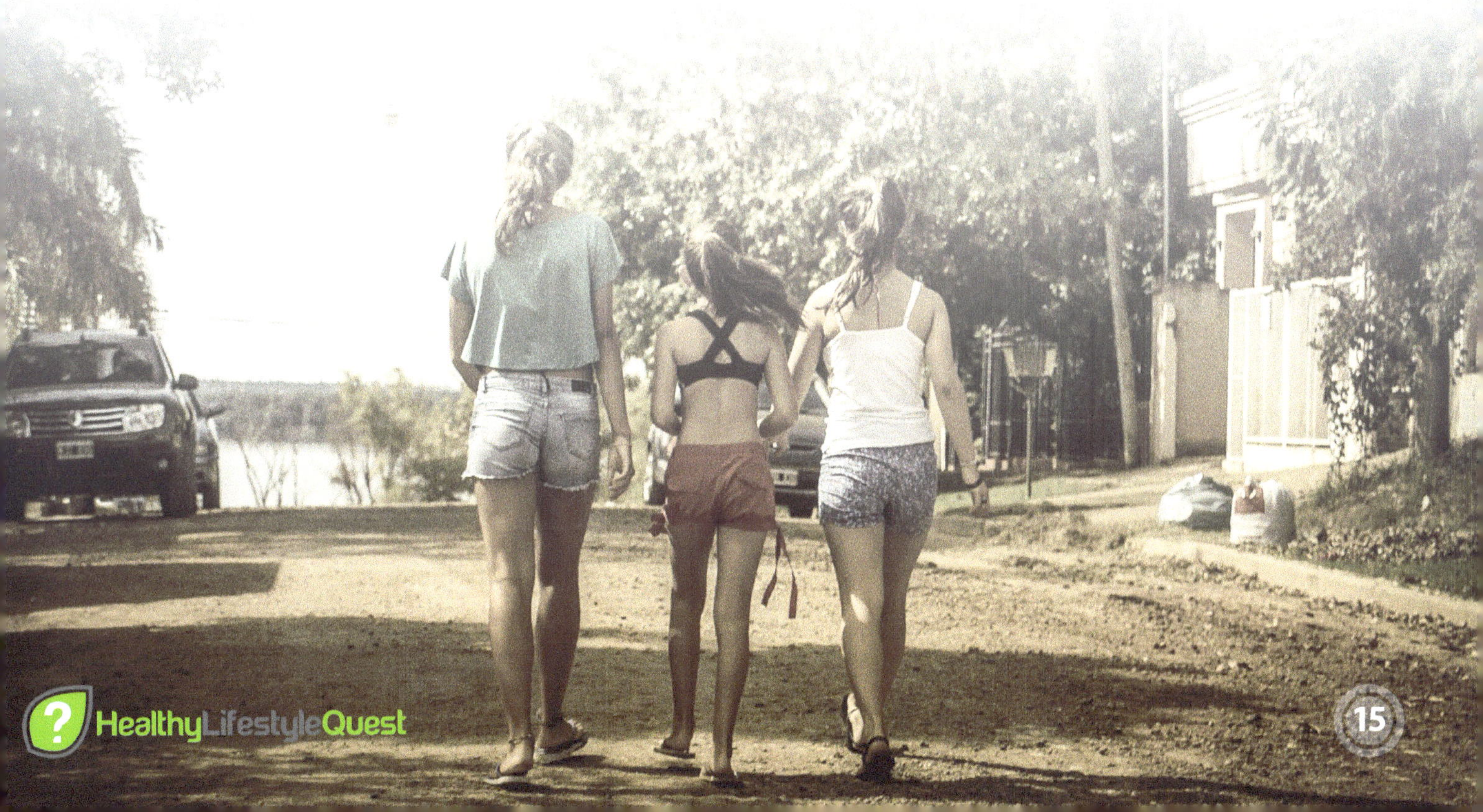

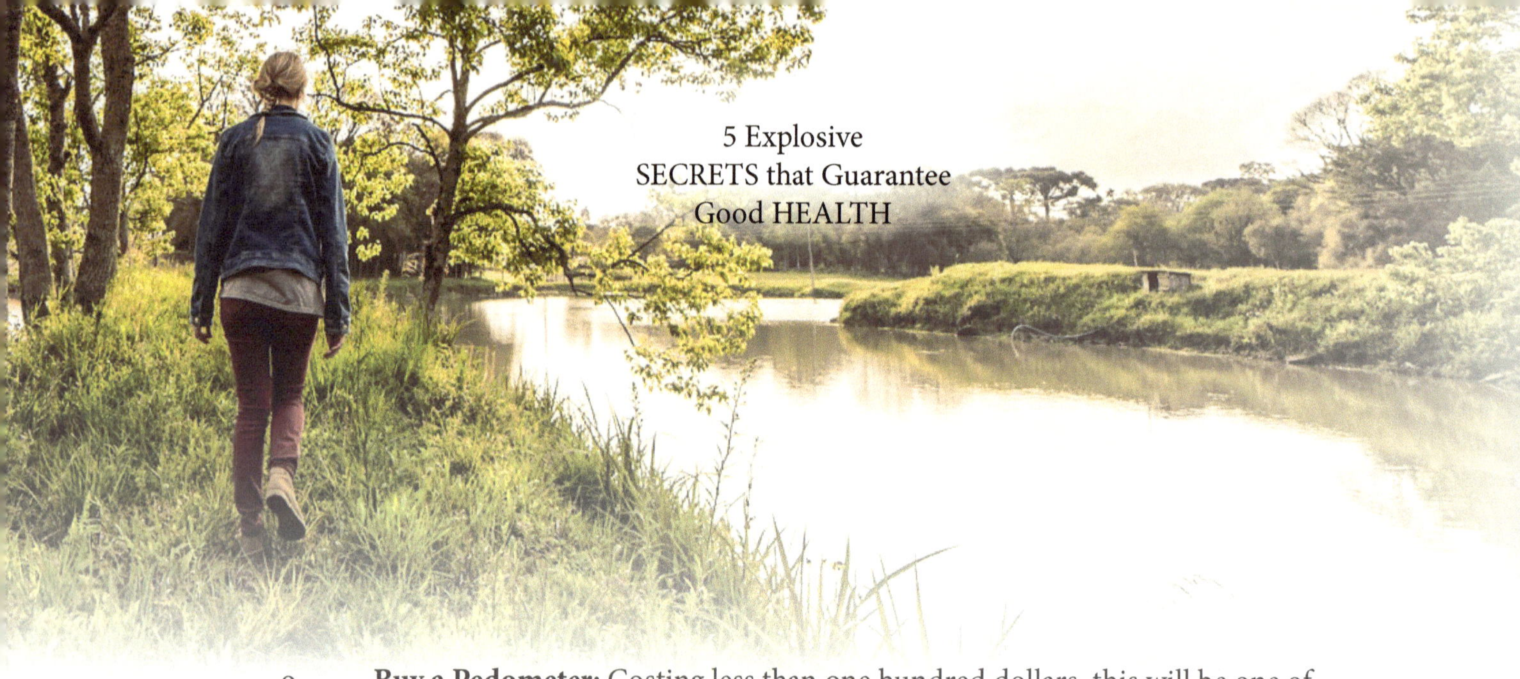


o        **Buy a Pedometer:** Costing less than one hundred dollars, this will be one of the most valuable investments within that price range for you.

o        **Use a Timer:** Simply use a timer to remind you of a pre-determined exercise routine. This may be a brief walk around the office building or even around your office. It does not have to be exotic, just a few simple body movement to get the stiffness out of your muscles and ensure that you are closer to meeting your daily walk quota.

o        **Make Use of an Exercise Ball:** As a word of caution, you should not use this as a replacement for walking. The advantage this offers you is the opportunity to quickly execute a few exercises even while working. Of course, it also improve your balance and flexibility.

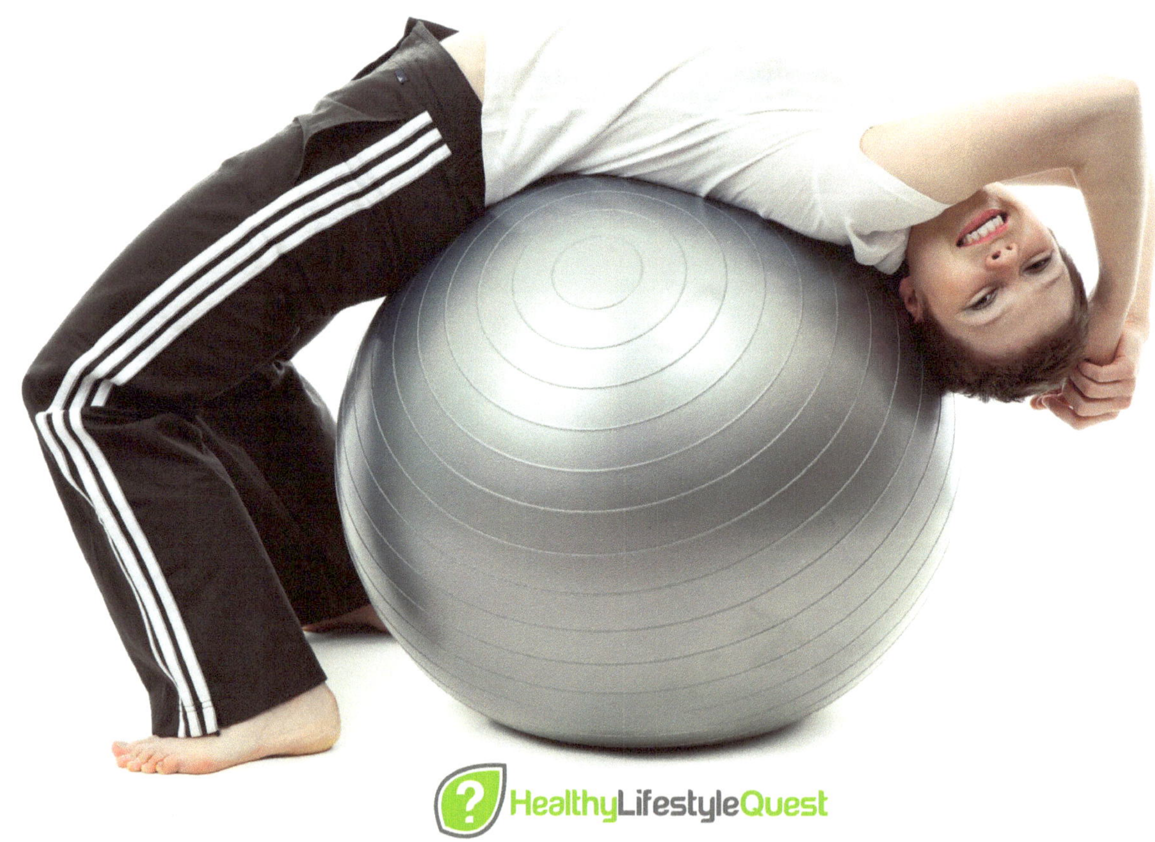

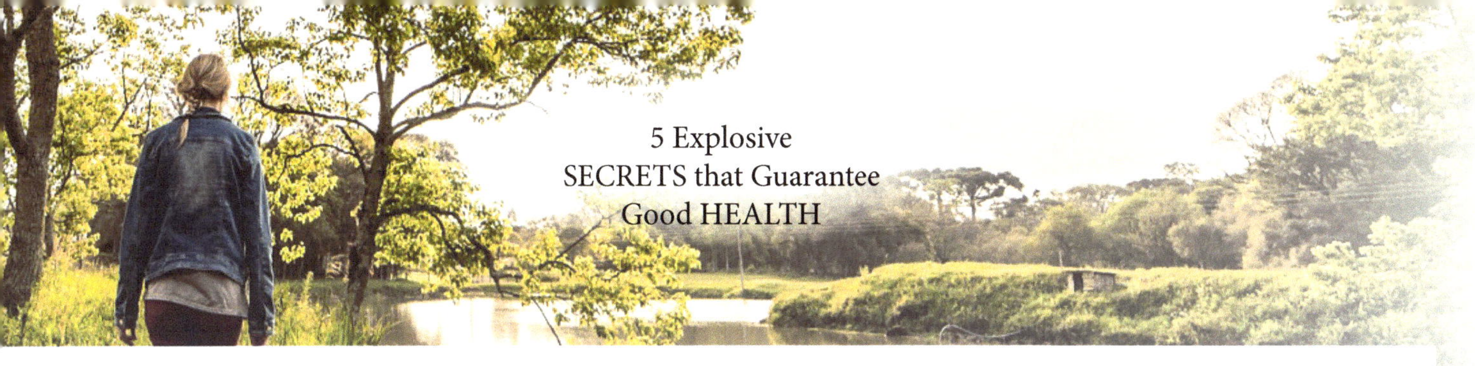


# Understanding HIIT, Exercise and Cardio

**High Intensity Interval Training (HIIT)** is one of the novel exercise routines rapidly gaining popularity due to its well-touted benefits.

It entails carrying out high intensity exercise routines between periods of moderate rest.

**Its highly intense combination makes it suitable for execution a maximum of three** times a week.

**Studies have shown that HIIT practiced over twelve weeks could result in notable reductions in total abdominal, trunk as well as visceral fat. It is well suited to people who have tight schedules yet desire to keep fit optimally.**

According to the American College of Sports Medicine, cardiovascular fitness refers to the ability of the body to receive, transport and utilize oxygen while carrying out exercises. It is only able to do this when the heart, lungs, muscles and blood work together while you carry out your exercise routine. It is therefore a veritable yardstick for measuring the soundness of your health.

**A sedentary lifestyle has practically no benefits for anyone. You must get your body moving in order to derive maximum benefits from it and its functions.**

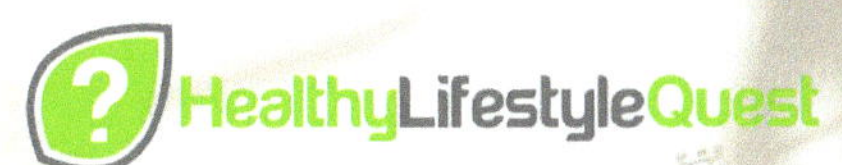

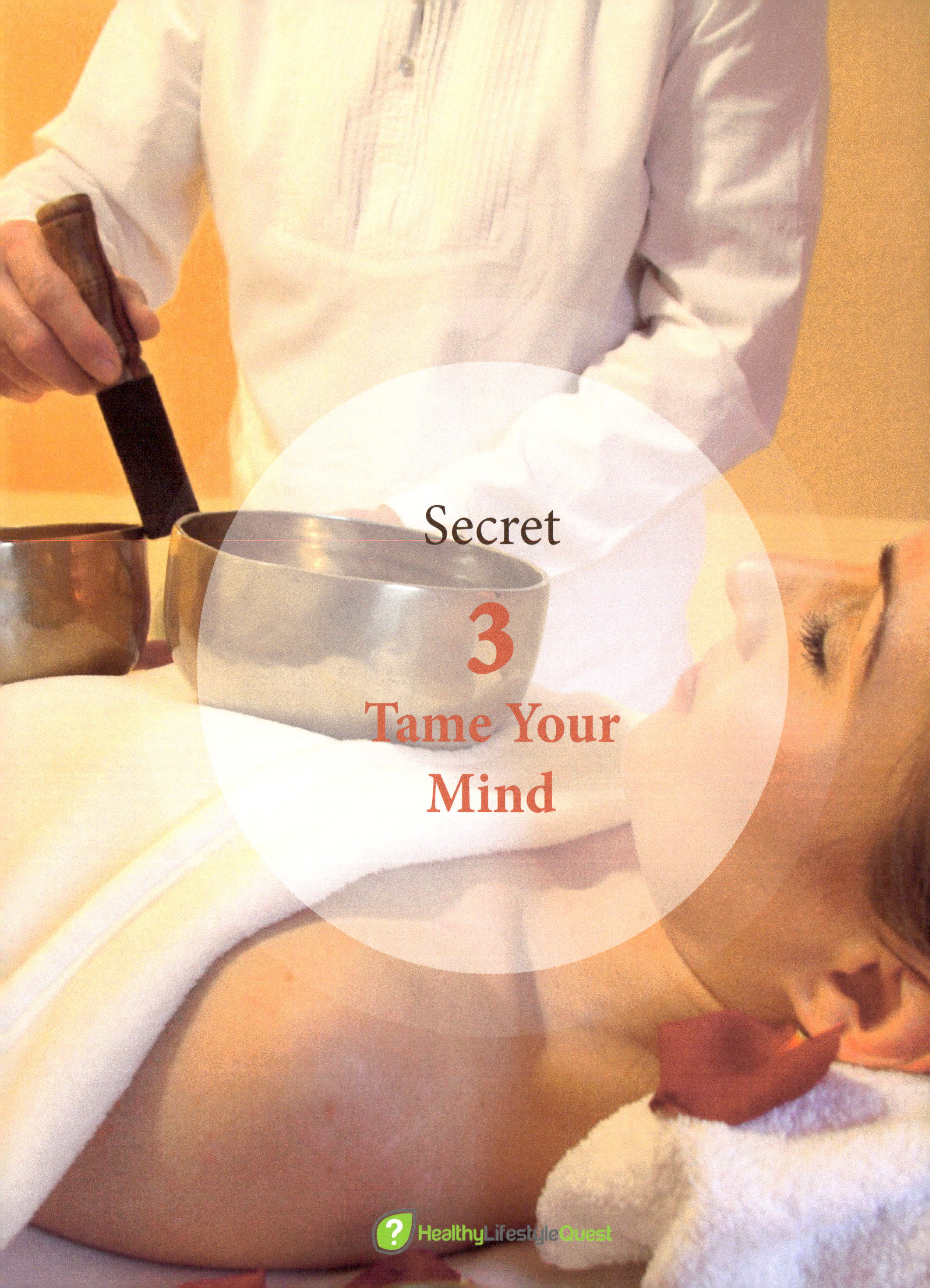
Secret
3
Tame Your
Mind
HealthyLifestyleQuest

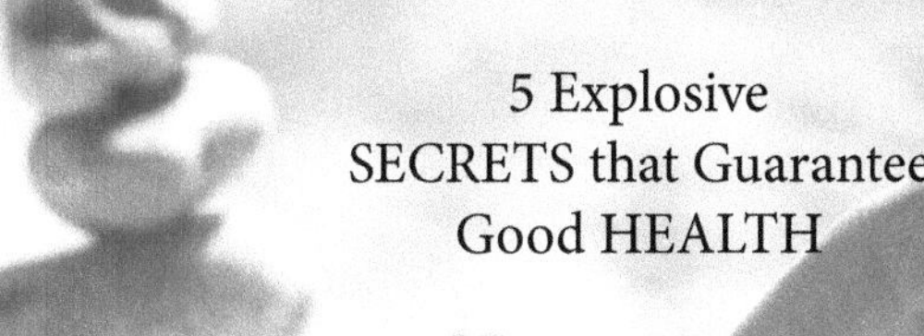


# How does the mind affect the body?

**This question always rises to the fore when most people hear about the mind-body relationship. Is there really a relationship?**

An estimated 40 million adults in the United States suffer from anxiety disorders. These anxiety disorders are a product of excessive worrying. Most people actually carry a lot repressed feelings such as denied grief, emotional pain, anger and trauma and these feelings are embedded in the cells of the bodies with the common manifestation being migraine headache, ache in the lower back region of the body, high blood pressure or stomach ulcer.

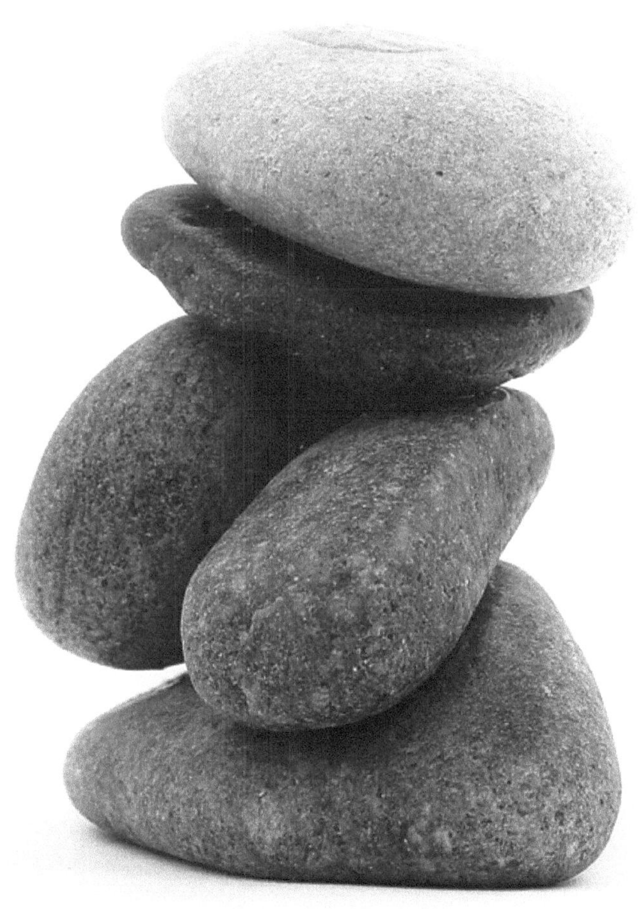

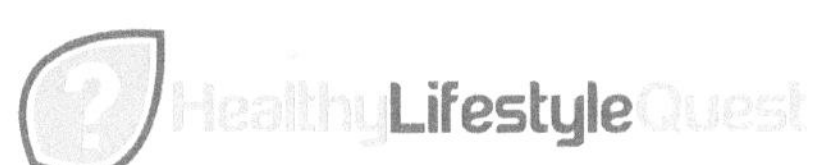

# Improving Your Emotional Health

**Knowing this, it is critical to closely monitor your emotional health. What are the risks of possessing negative emotional health?**

Here are a few…

o **Weakening of Body's Immune System:** The human body cannot cope with a regular dosage of negative emotion. It is bound to cave in at some point. The danger here is the fallout which is typically a series of physical ailments resulting from the weakened immune system that prevents the body from fighting as it normally should. Infections find it easy to set it and cause damage to the body at this stage.

o **Drug Abuse:** Inasmuch as the human body may be weakened from negative emotional health, it can also try artificial means of resolving its shortfall in natural strength. Such means include use of unprescribed medications and outright abuse of drugs. Alcohol and tobacco consumption could also increase at this stage.

o **Regular Illnesses:** Negative emotional health creates a doorway for illnesses to set in and even flourish.  These include back pain, headaches, insomnia, stomach upset, palpitations and constipation among many others.

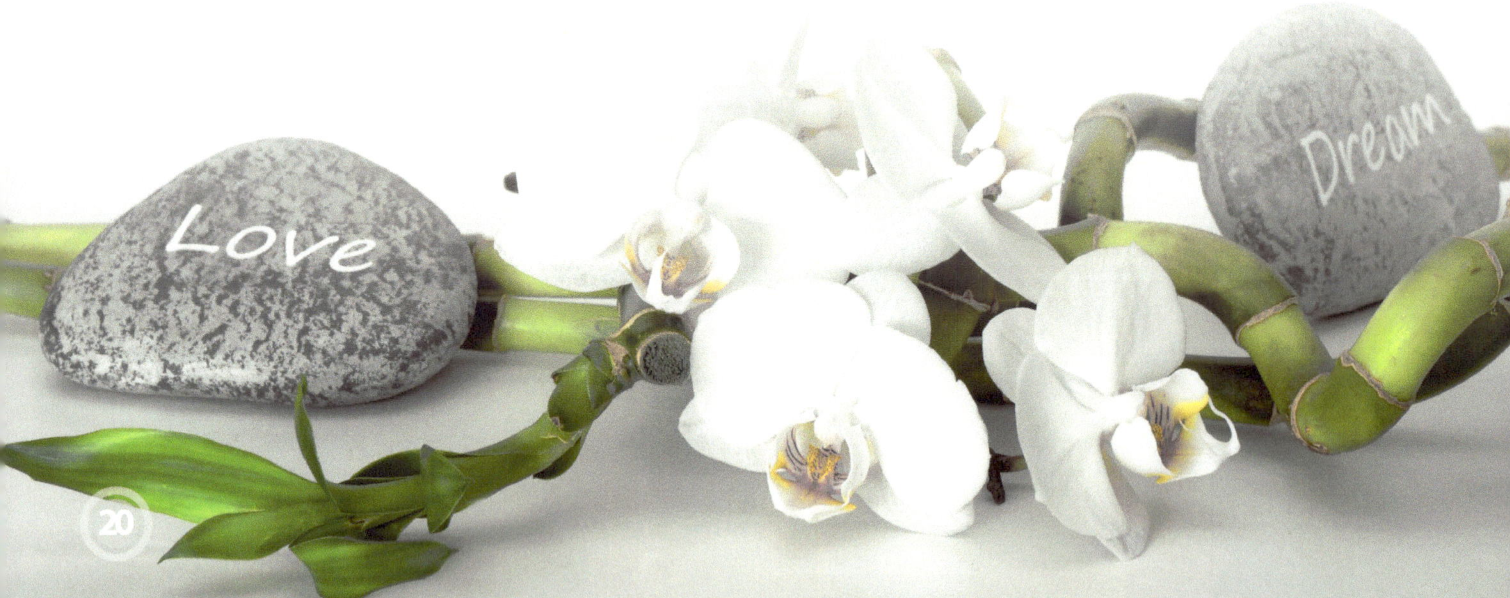

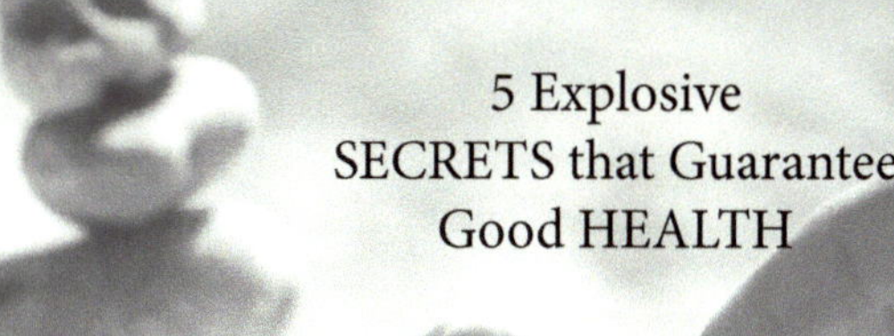


# Benefits of Positive Emotional Health

Having seen the damage that may be caused by negative emotional health, we will now take a look at the other side of the coin.

These include:

o **Feeling of Contentment:** People who are mentally healthy tend to feel contented with their environment and most people around them.

o **Feeling of Meaning and Purpose in Life:** These people are able to find some meaning in life and maintain meaningful relationships.

o **High Self-confidence and Esteem:** Being mentally healthy enables an individual to build high self-esteem and confidence. This translates to the ability to take initiative and accomplish meaningful goals in life.

o **Zestful Living:** This is like a feedback loop. As you exhibit positive mental health, life becomes more enjoyable thus enabling you to exude more characteristics of positive emotional health. It works its way around continuously.

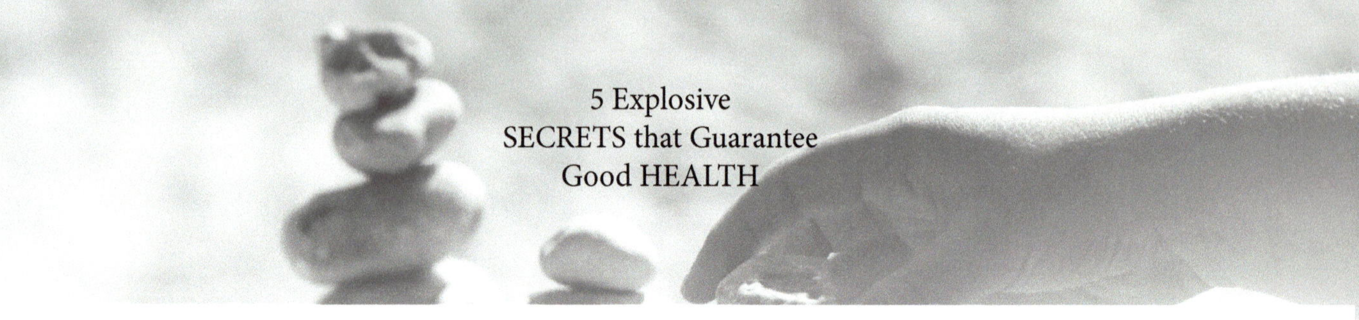


# Living a Happy, Stress-free and Relaxed Life...while Remaining Busy!

**If you currently have the mindset that being busy means being unhappy, get ready to ditch that notion with these five easy tips.**

o        **Express Yourself Appropriately:** Bottling up feelings inside of you will not do any good. Examples of such destructive feelings include sadness and anxiety. Who do you talk to? Of course, family members are typically the first you would approach but you must also know that in certain situation, you have to seek professional help. These may be from psychologists, doctors and religious advisors. At the end, you may receive counsel or professional advice that will provide the right turnaround to your emotional health.

o        **Calm Your Mind:** It is not your mind alone that needs to be calmed. The body also needs to be calmed and this can be achieved via meditation and other methods such as simple exercises. Examples of meditation techniques include Yoga and Tai Chi.

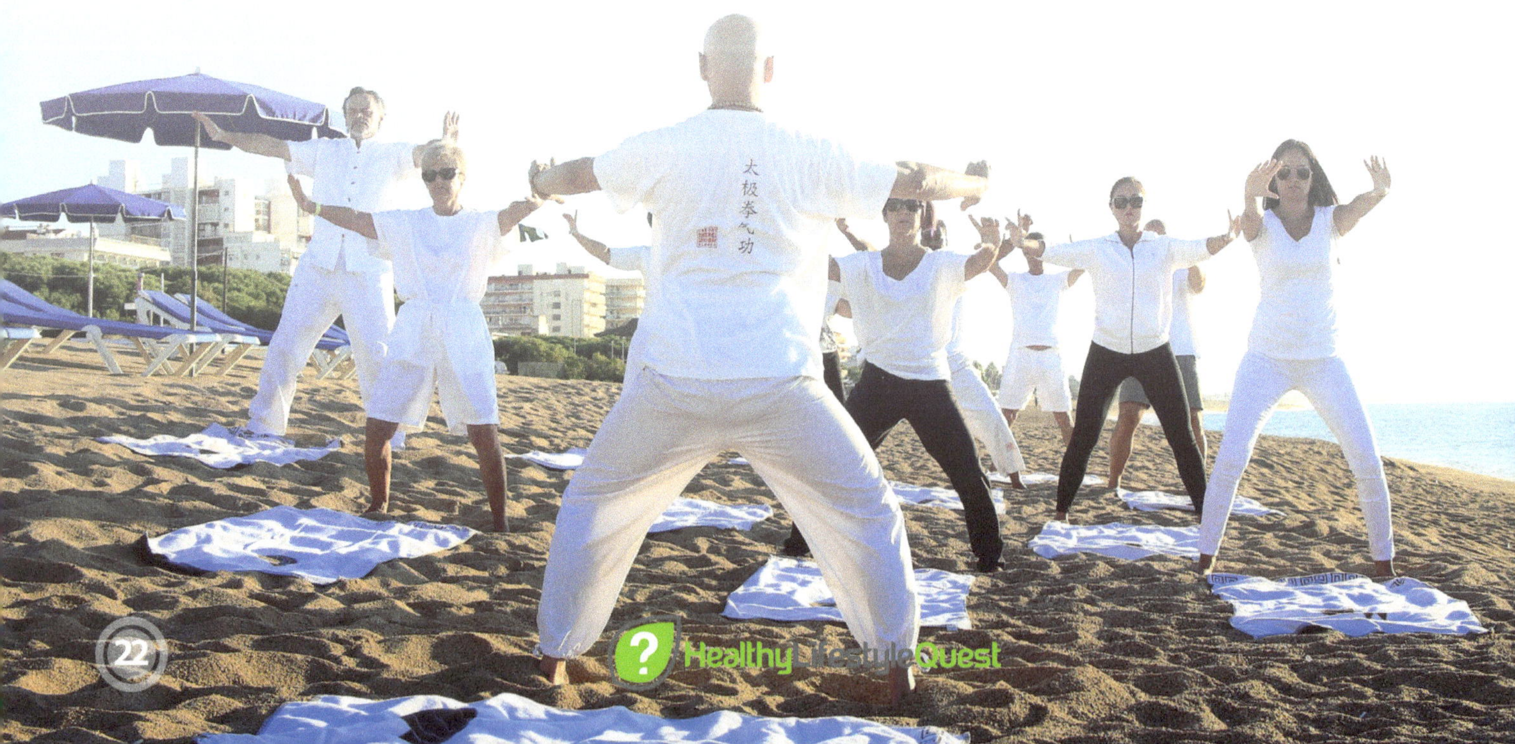

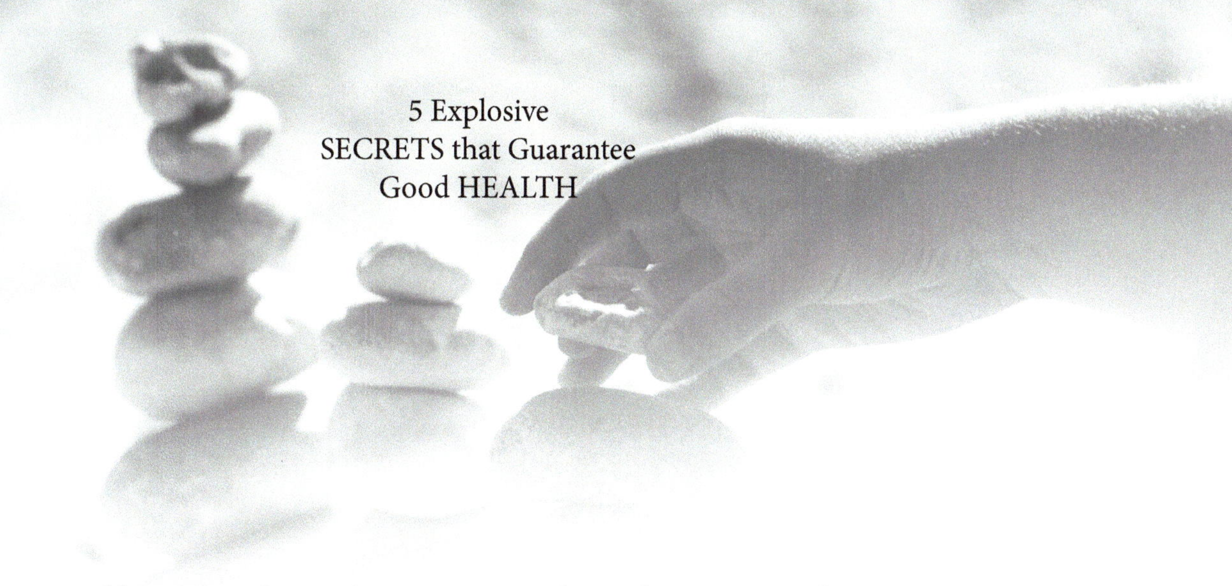


o       **Build Strong Relationships:** Negative relationships are typical stressors. On the other hand, positive relationships are a source of emotional release and upliftment. It is very important to build the latter kind of relationships so that you can rely on them when difficulties arise.

o       **Develop a Resilient Character:** It is important to develop a character that will withstand life's curveballs. Drawing up strategies to combat diverse situations is a great way of acting proactively to cheat negative emotional health.

o       **Live a Balanced Life:** As tempting as it is to remain on a particular lane throughout life, ensuring that your office and home lives are separate is very important. Enjoy the best of both but make sure the two lanes don't intersect and cause a traffic jam for either or both!

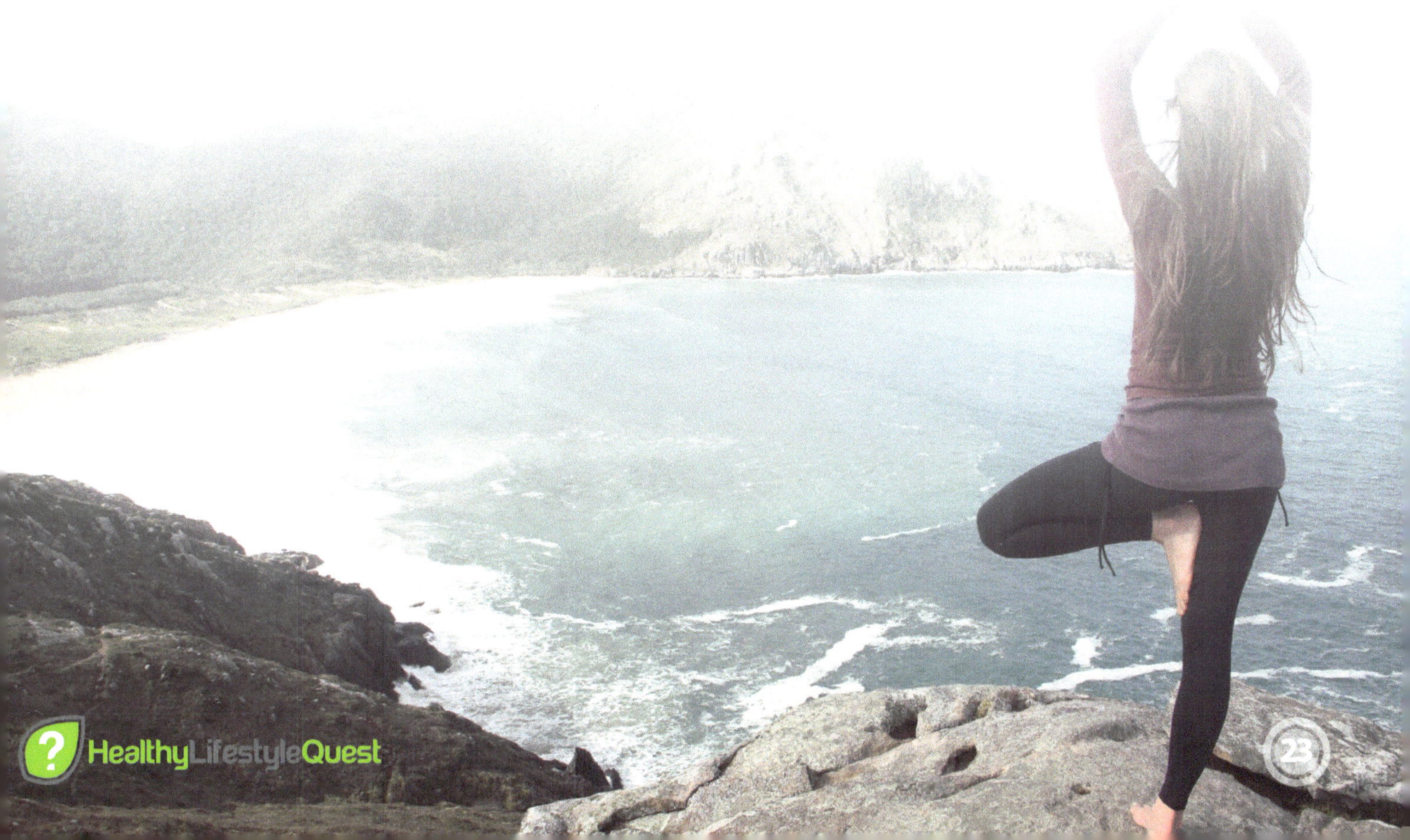

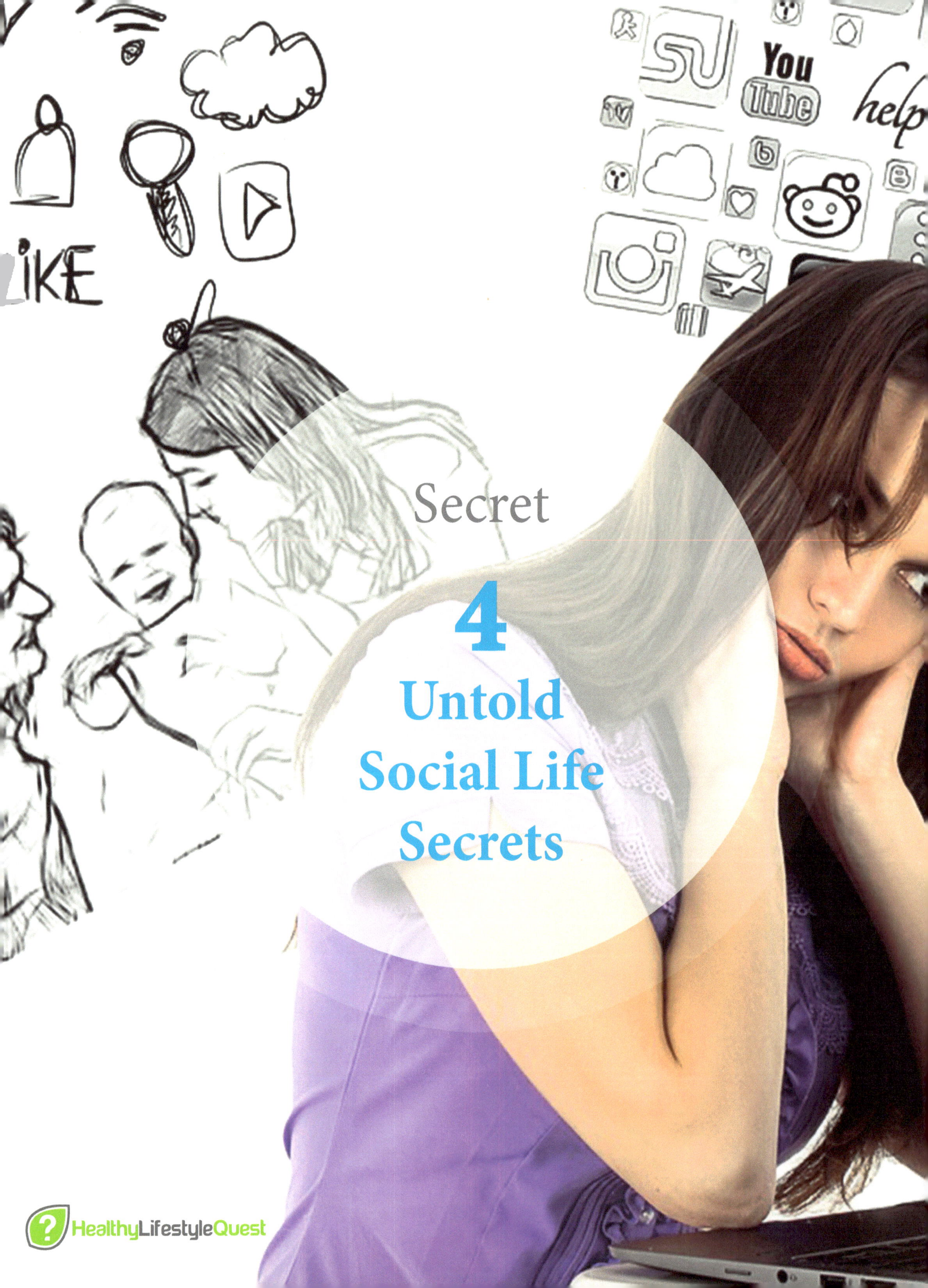

LIKE
Secret
4
Untold
Social Life
Secrets
HealthyLifestyleQuest

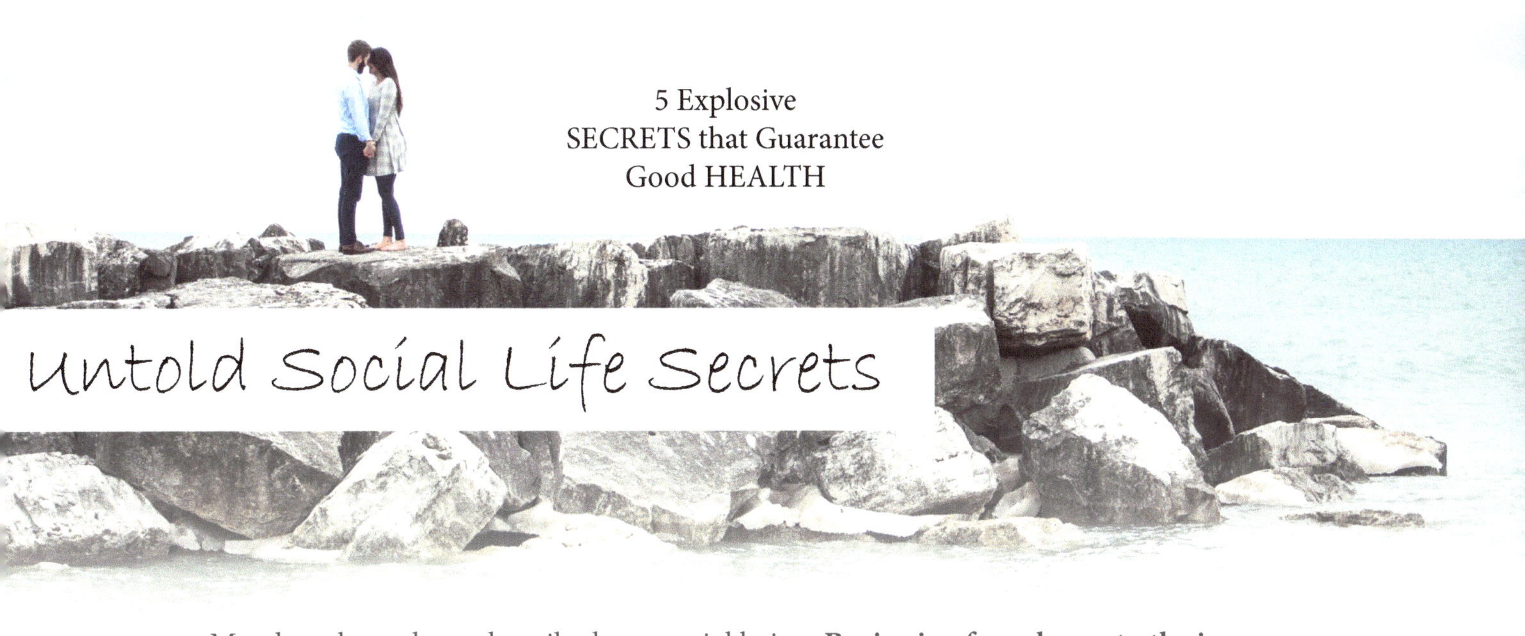


# Untold Social Life Secrets

Man has always been described as a social being. **Beginning from home to the immediate surroundings and larger society, you is constantly being influenced by the events and people around you.**

The resultant effect on your health is profound as both factors may be grouped either as stressors or invigorators. While circumstances may determine which group a person or event may fall under, the individual also plays a role.

How do you perceive people and events? Do you react negatively to adverse circumstances? Having dealt with emotional health previously, it becomes very easy for you to see the thread running through these otherwise separate factors.

As you interact with people and experience events around you, it is difficult to remain the same as your reaction to both will determine your emotional state which will in turn determine how healthy you will be.

It is clear that the interrelationship between you, society and your relations with people provides the basis for a balanced health. The question therefore is, how are you dealing with both factors?

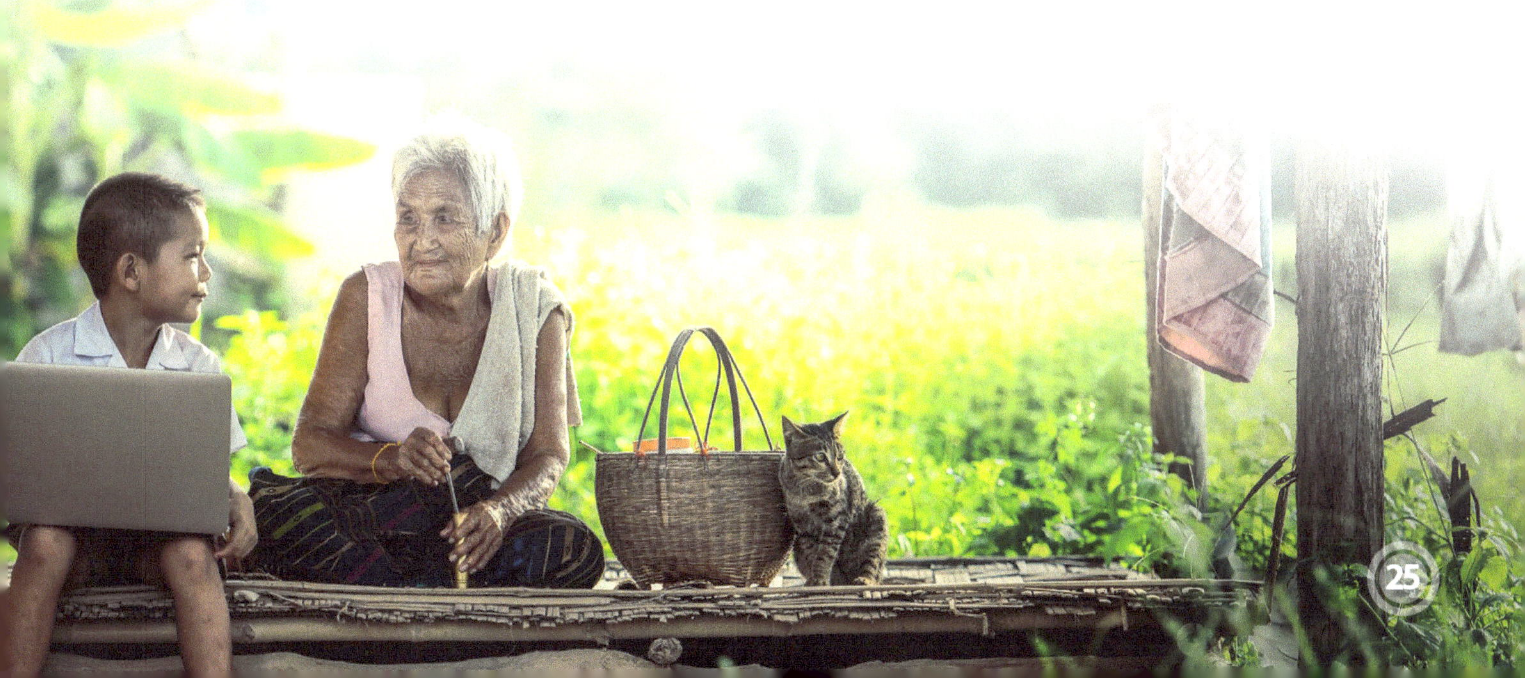

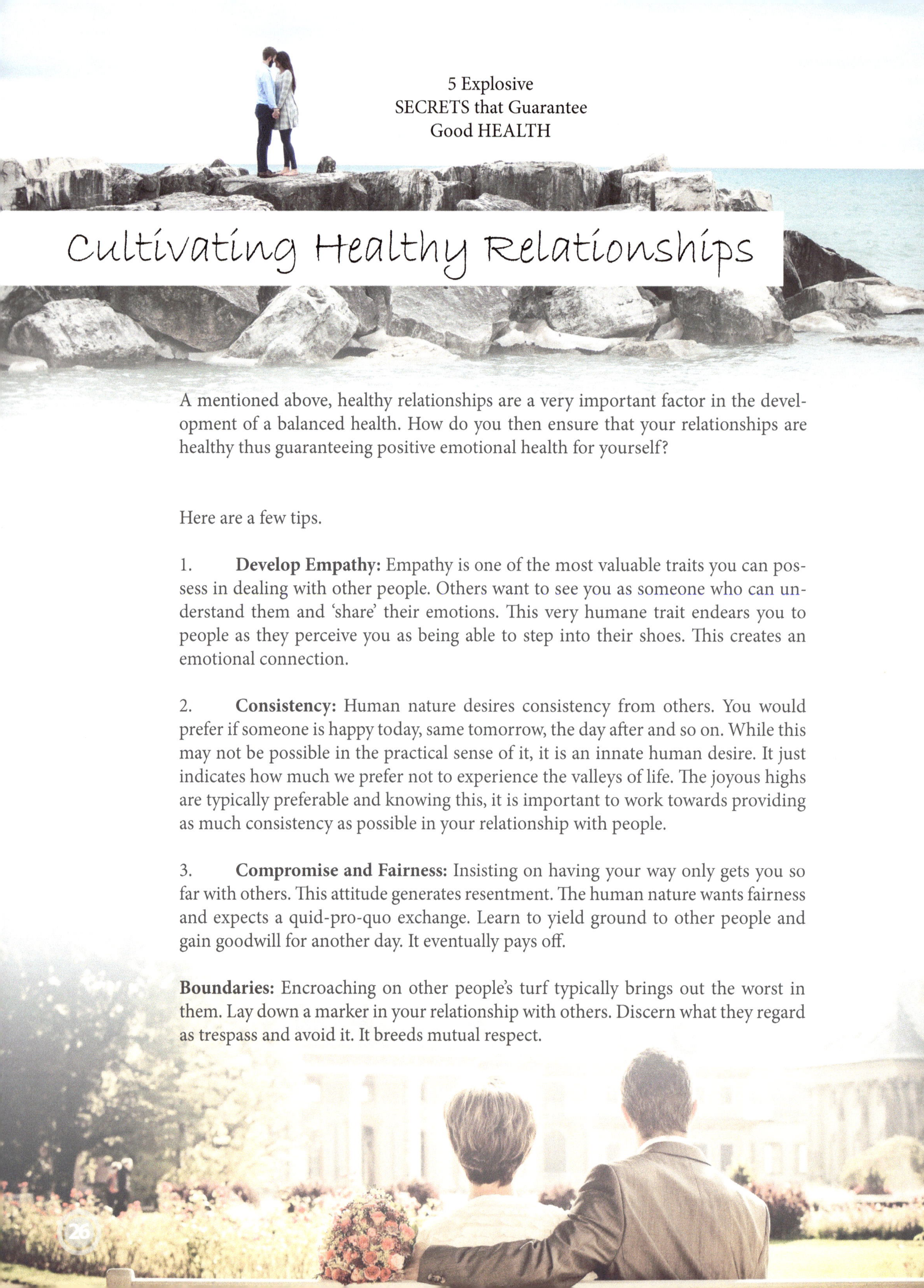


# Cultivating Healthy Relationships

A mentioned above, healthy relationships are a very important factor in the development of a balanced health. How do you then ensure that your relationships are healthy thus guaranteeing positive emotional health for yourself?

Here are a few tips.

1.    **Develop Empathy:** Empathy is one of the most valuable traits you can possess in dealing with other people. Others want to see you as someone who can understand them and 'share' their emotions. This very humane trait endears you to people as they perceive you as being able to step into their shoes. This creates an emotional connection.

2.    **Consistency:** Human nature desires consistency from others. You would prefer if someone is happy today, same tomorrow, the day after and so on. While this may not be possible in the practical sense of it, it is an innate human desire. It just indicates how much we prefer not to experience the valleys of life. The joyous highs are typically preferable and knowing this, it is important to work towards providing as much consistency as possible in your relationship with people.

3.    **Compromise and Fairness:** Insisting on having your way only gets you so far with others. This attitude generates resentment. The human nature wants fairness and expects a quid-pro-quo exchange. Learn to yield ground to other people and gain goodwill for another day. It eventually pays off.

**Boundaries:** Encroaching on other people's turf typically brings out the worst in them. Lay down a marker in your relationship with others. Discern what they regard as trespass and avoid it. It breeds mutual respect.

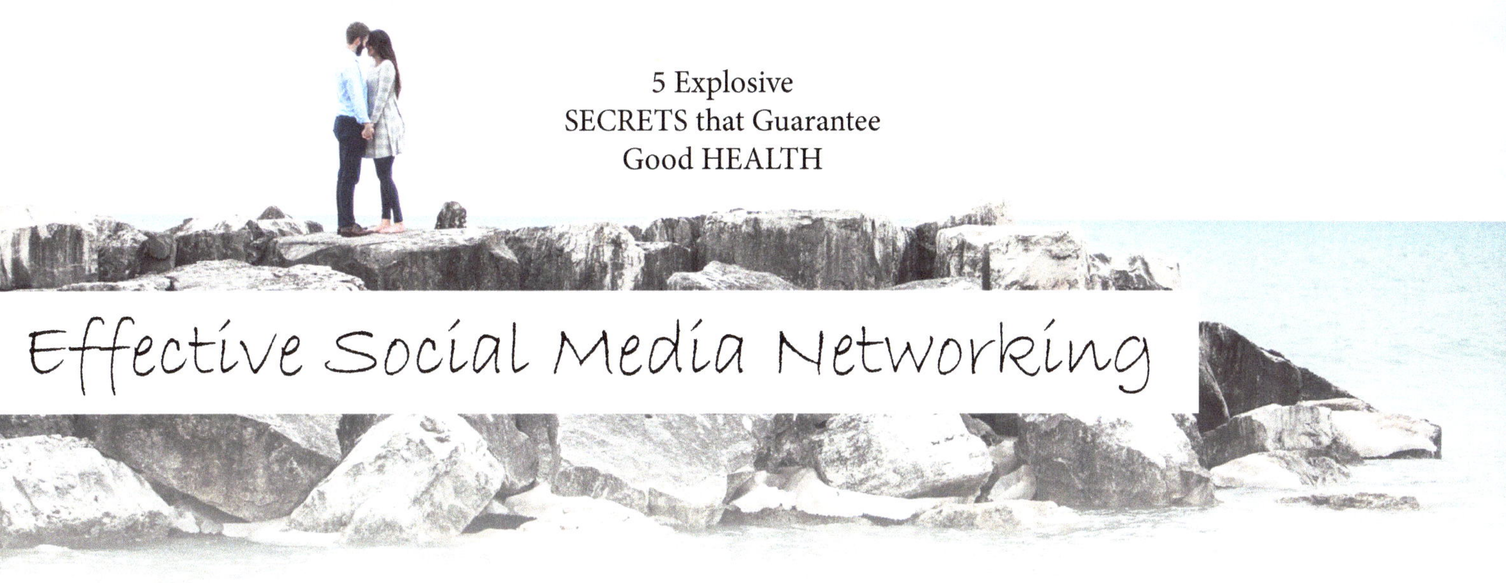


# Effective Social Media Networking

It looks like the alternate universe; the social media galaxy seems to spot many channels that allow you to connect with others in a virtual society.

We have mentioned relationships mostly in the physical sense of it but in contemporary times, the virtual world competes with the physical. The reality however, is that relationship rules differ in some instances between the two worlds.

**How can you effectively network on social media, make friends, build strong relationships and have positive emotional health translating to good health balance?**

These few tips should help:

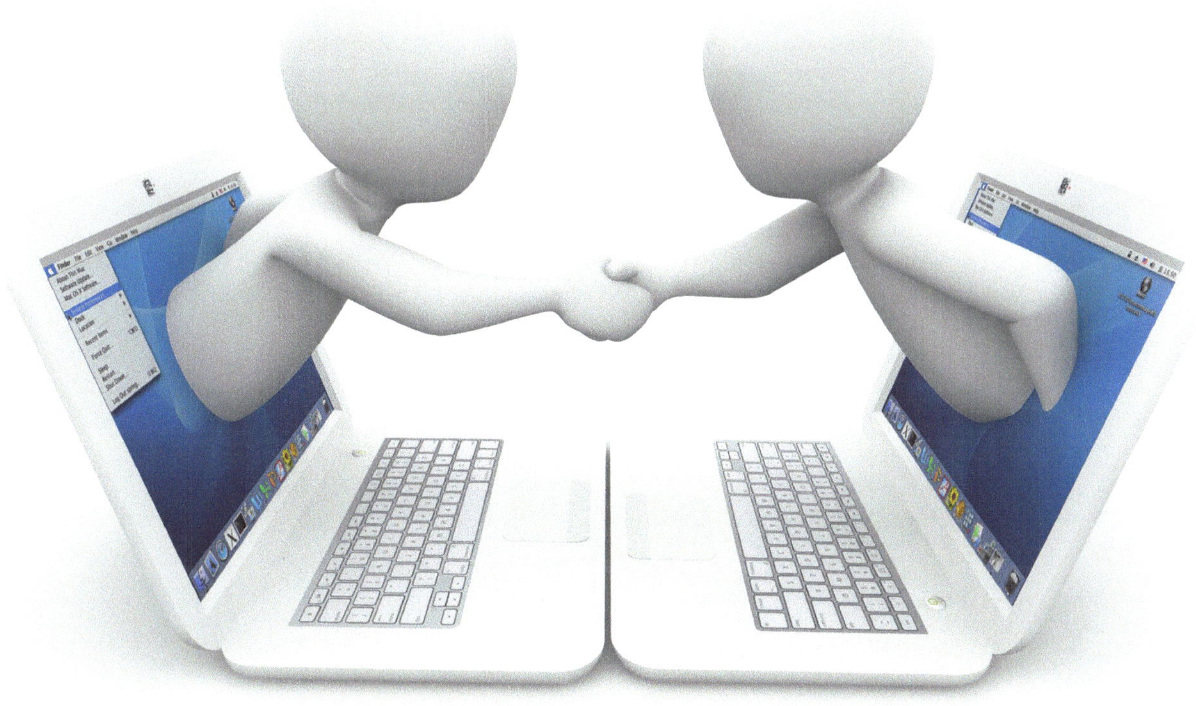

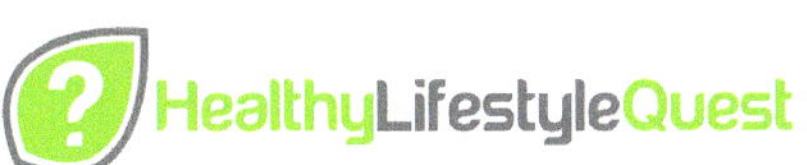

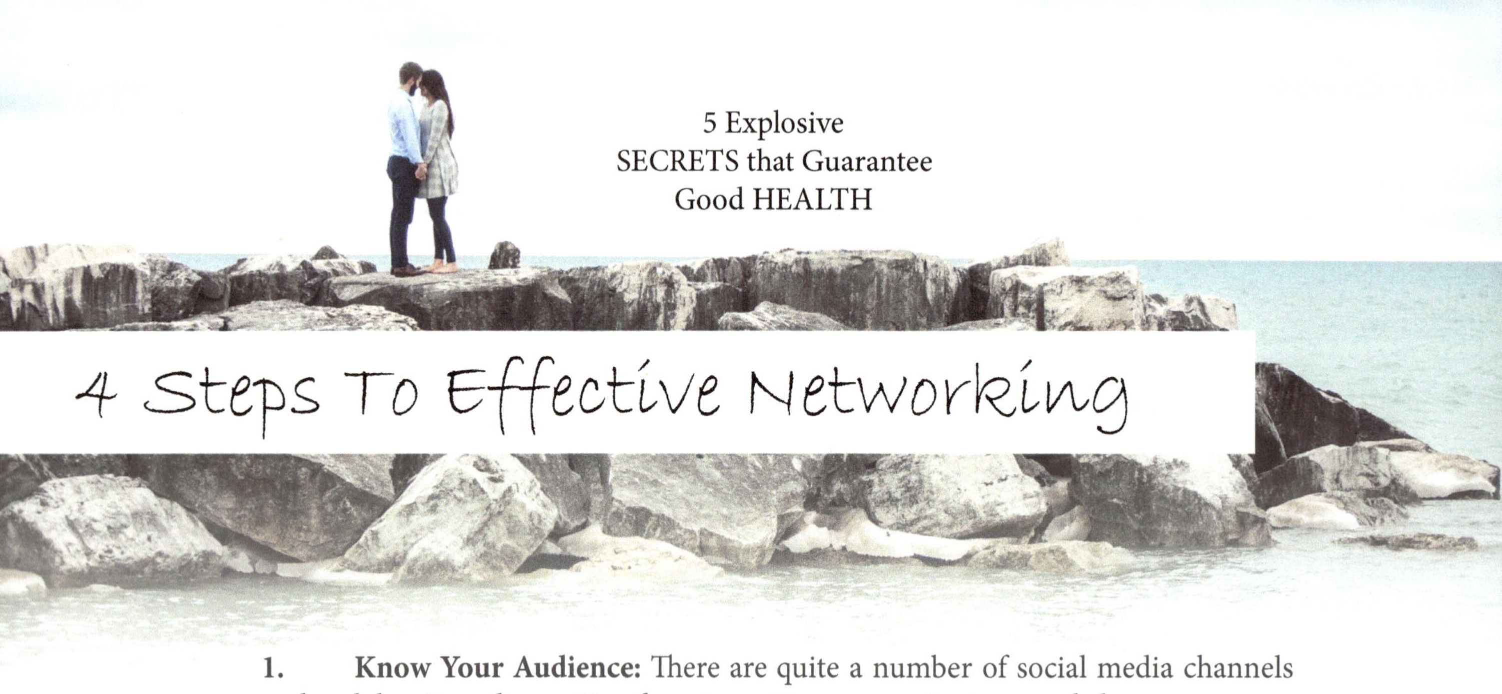


# 4 Steps To Effective Networking

1.      **Know Your Audience:** There are quite a number of social media channels and each has its audience. You do not want to communicate wrongly because you are not with the right crowd.

2.      **Choose Your Channels:** Having a profile on every network may sound like a nice idea but do you really need to? It is important to focus on the primary channels that fulfill your purpose of being on social media. This will ensure that you derive maximum value from your networking efforts.

3.      **Maintain a Clean Profile:** Avoid the doubtful profiles that populate many social media channels today. Go 'green' with a profile that projects a positive image. You want to attract the best friends and build strong relationship? It begins with a clean profile.

4.  **Contribute Meaningfully:** The most important factor in effective networking on social media is meaningful contribution. This may vary in context from one channel to another but the principle remains the same. Provide value and you will gain reciprocal respect.

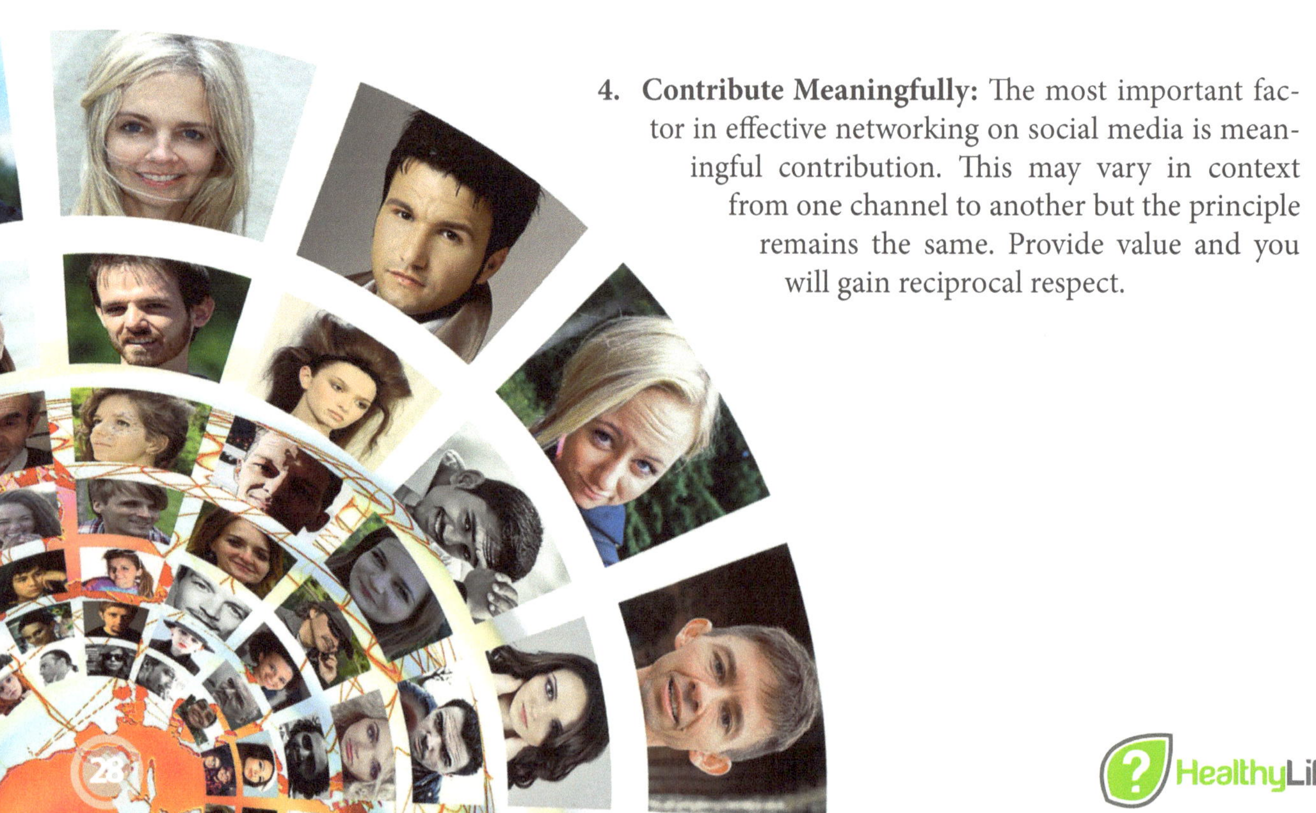



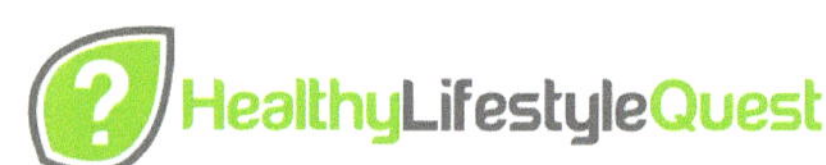

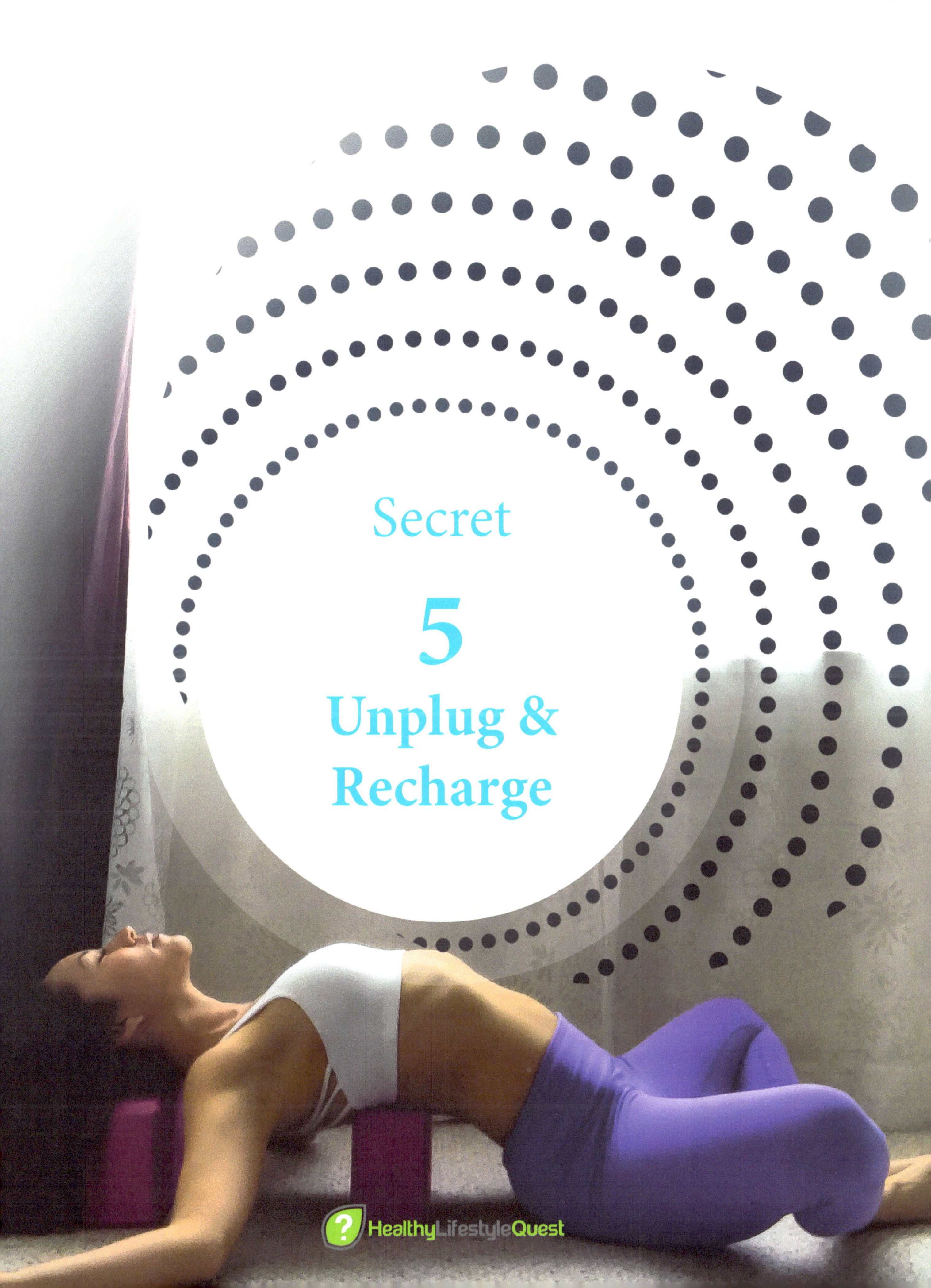
Secret

5

Unplug &
Recharge

HealthyLifestyleQuest

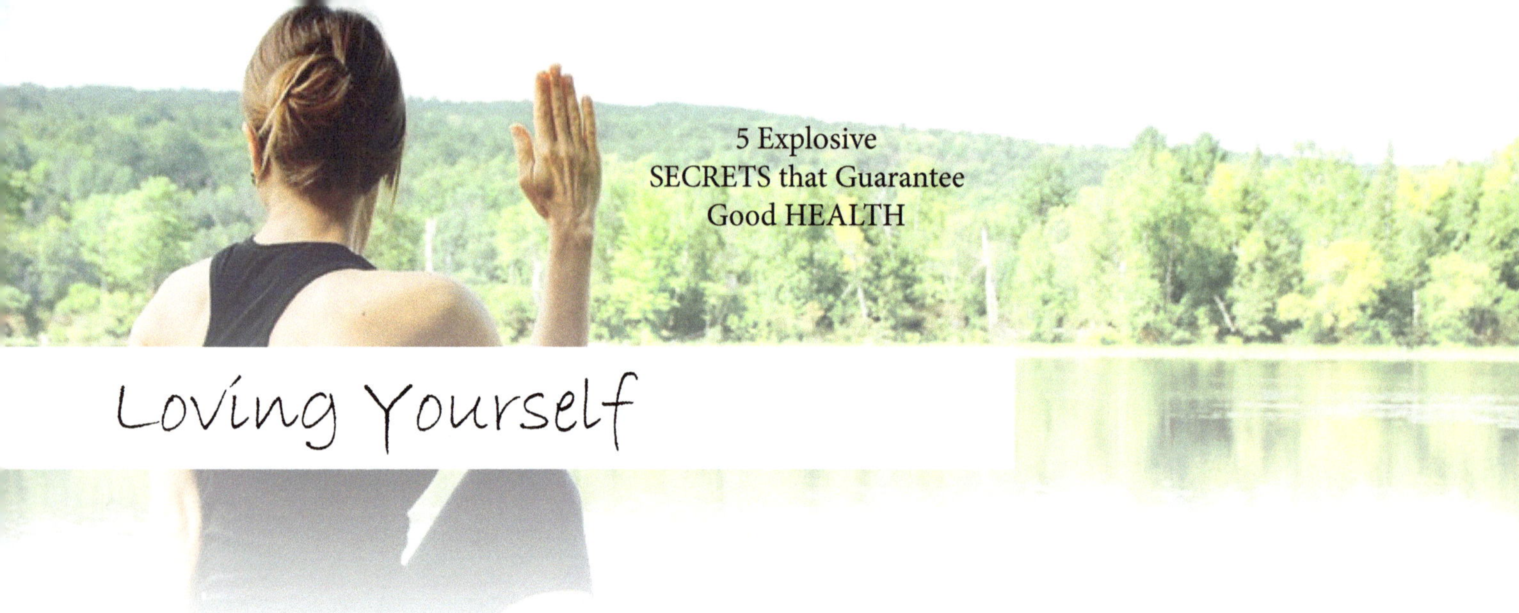


# Loving Yourself

**Do you love yourself? Of course you do!**
Do you show that love to yourself in practical terms? You ask how?

Well, these are just a few ways you may prove your love to yourself.

1.      **Proper Rest:** The human body was not designed to do physical labor round the clock, all year round. It actually has provision for adequate rest and when that requirement is not fulfilled, it could lead (and often does) to a health crisis. Want to show your body some love? First step is proper rest.

2.      **Spare Time for Yourself:** Most people think of outings in terms of pairings or groupings. However, this is mere convention as nothing restrains you from treating yourself to a vacation, movie, art exhibition or music concert among others. Learn to create that time for yourself to have fun and loosen up.

**How does all this pay off?**
You get to experience joy and lightheartedness. You free your mind of unnecessary load, connect with people around you and experience new places. Ultimately, you have positive emotional health and optimum physical health to go with it.

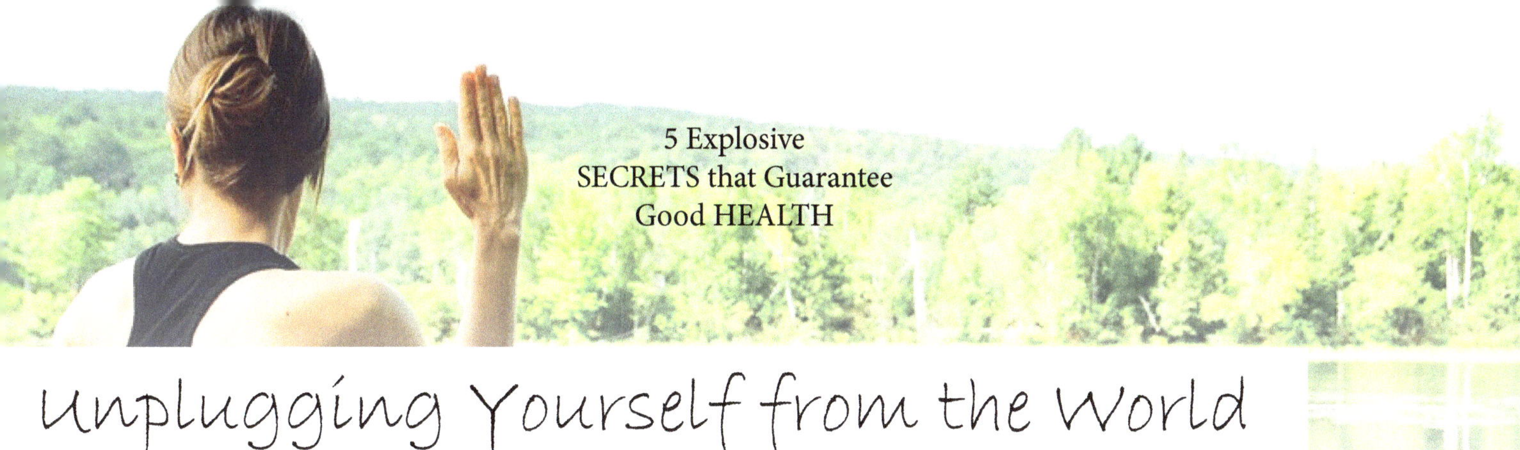


# Unplugging Yourself from the World

There are times when you just want to stop all activities and do a full factory reset on yourself. You want to unclog the mental pores caked with everyday hassles and just get away from…everything. Everyone feels like that sometimes.

How do you achieve this? Read on…

o      Take a vacation

o      Write a book

o      Go bungee jumping

o      Visit a monastery

o      Switch off all phones for a week

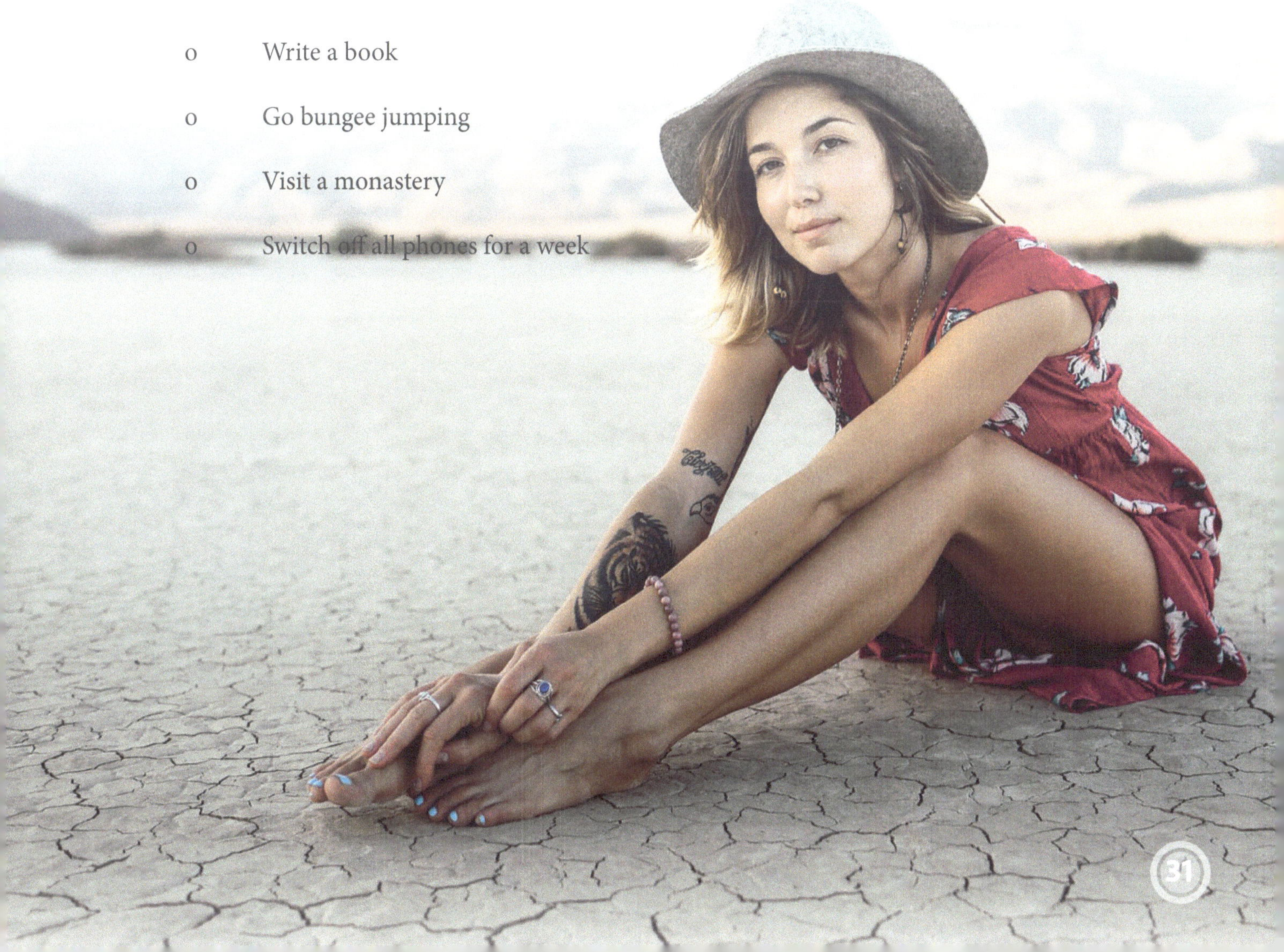

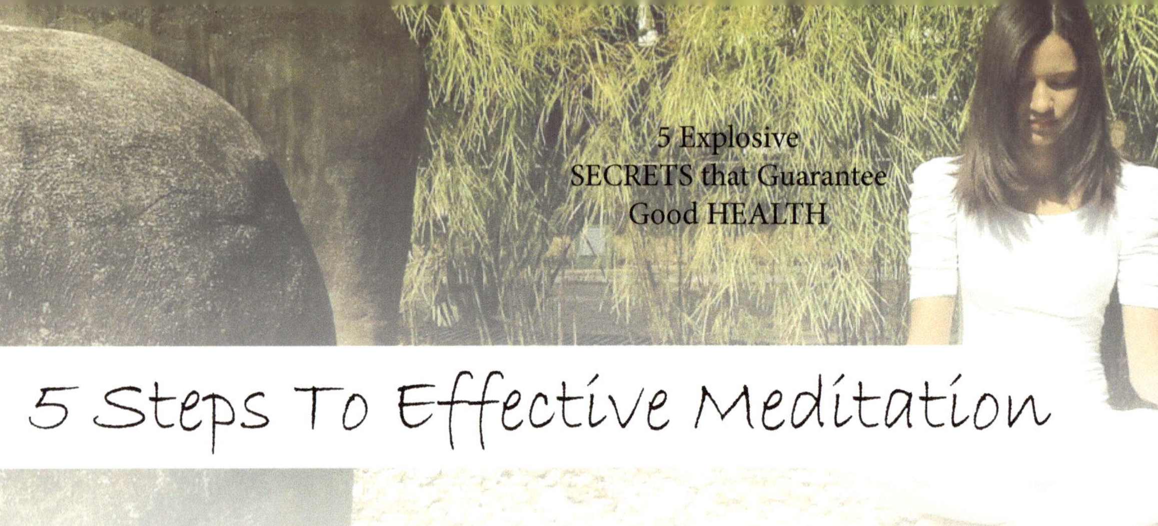


# 5 Steps To Effective Meditation

**One of the best ways to tale your mind off the world around you is to meditate.** This is easy to learn but requires practice to be of optimum use to you.

Here are a few steps...

1. **Find a Meditation Spot:** The more consistent you are with this, the better on the long run. It should be away from public eye. Privacy is important in meditation.

2. **Assume Comfortable Position:** There are diverse positions for meditation. The key factor however, is comfort.

3. **Clear Your Mind:** Meditation is of no use to you if your mind is clogged with issues of day to day life. You must consciously empty your mind of all thoughts and expect to receive a peaceful feeling in replacement as you enter into meditation. However, that is not as simple as it sounds. Beginners should start with guided meditation.

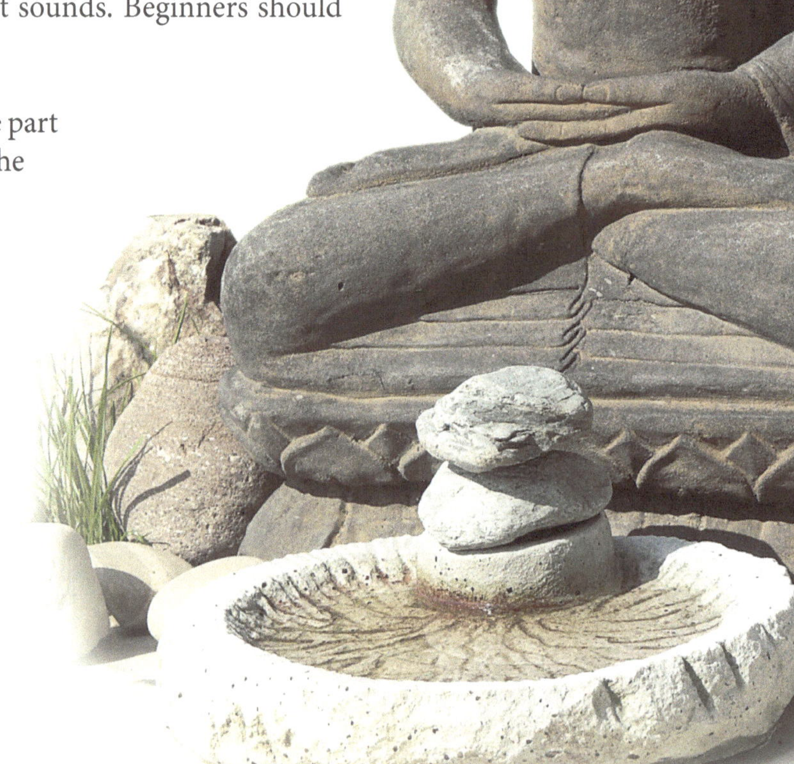

4. **Sit and Observe:** This is the part where you begin to experience the feeling of peace. Allow your mind flood with peaceful thoughts without pushing yourself in any direction deliberately. Just allow the peace flow.

5. **End the Meditation:** You simply ease out of it slowly. Don't just end abruptly and eject yourself mentally. Go with the flow. Ease out slowly.

# Conclusion

**Health is wealth.**

Thus goes the old yet evergreen saying.

You should subscribe to it and imbibe its truth. **Treat yourself with love, honor your body and give your mind decent emotional diet.**

**The combination of a positive emotional health and balanced physical health is priceless.**

**Go for it!**

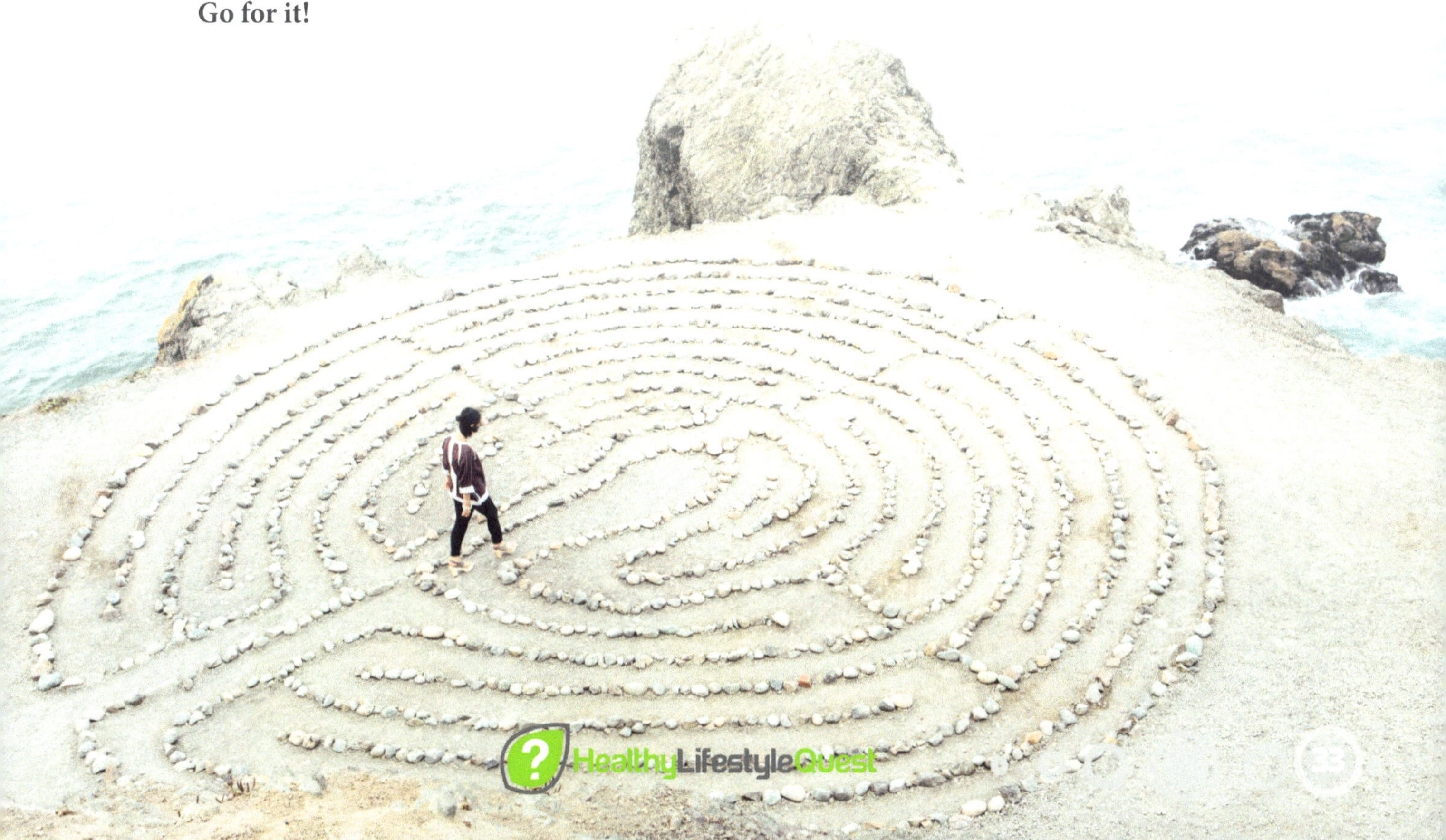

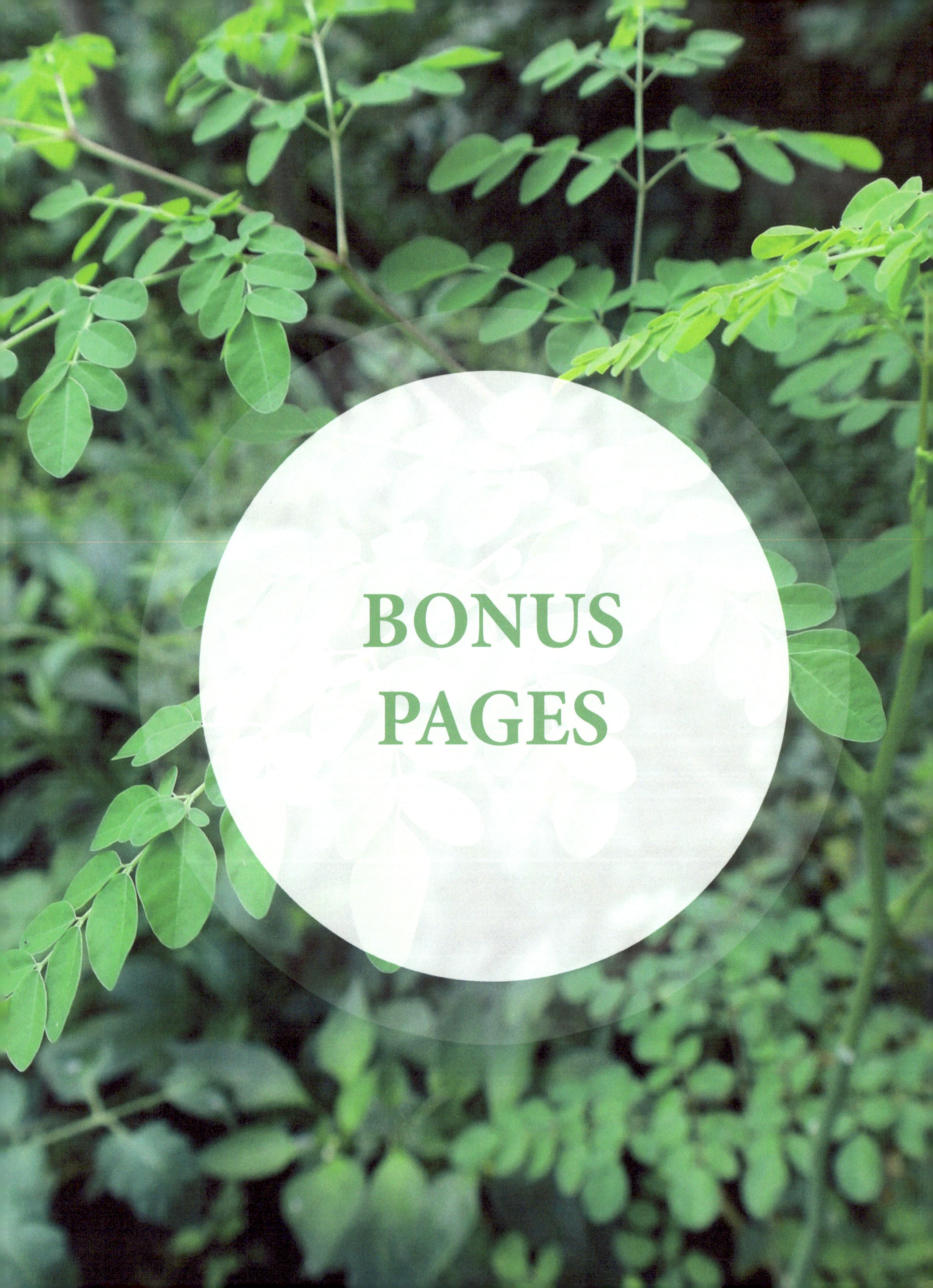
BONUS
PAGES

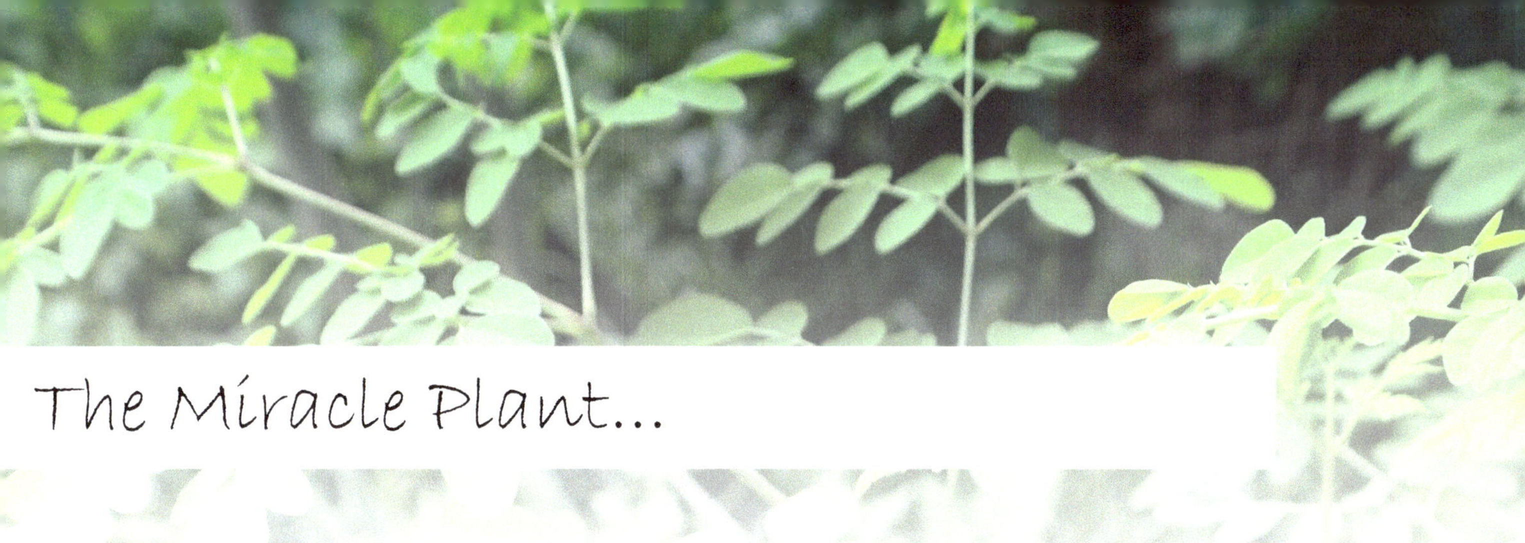

# The Miracle Plant...

If you're like most other people, each day you pop a multivitamin.

But did you know **there's a new superfood leaf more powerful than ANY multi-vitamin?**

Amazingly, thanks to its high concentration of the potent antioxidant, zeatin, <u>this leaf is bursting with anti-aging properties.</u>

According to the latest scientific research on nutrition and health, everyone who is currently taking a multivitamin could achieve exponentially better results by consuming this superfood instead.

(Cheap vitamin alternatives are likely stuffed full of fillers, binders, coatings, and artificial dyes that play havoc with your delicate system.)

What is this miracle plant?

**It's called Moringa.**

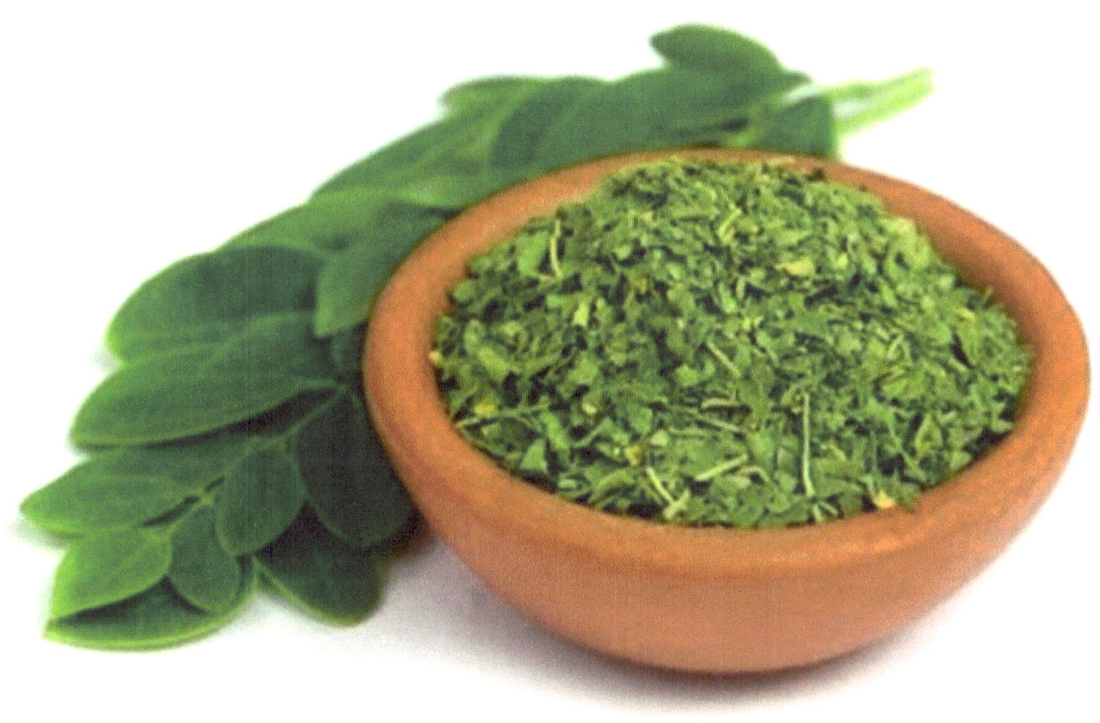

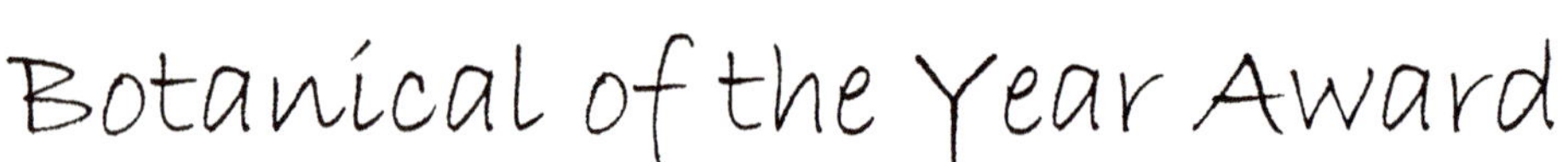

# Botanical of the Year Award

**It won the NIH's "Botanical of the Year" award because it's saved more lives in third world countries than any other plant.**

**<u>Truly, moringa is a super leaf.  It's been shown to…</u>**

Balance blood sugar levels…
Improve digestion
Strengthen the immune system…

Flush toxins from your liver…
Boost energy...
And lift your mood…

This mighty superfood leaf contains **<u>over ninety beneficial nutrients.</u>** A 100-gram serving of dry moringa leaf contains broad spectrum B vitamins, vitamin C, vitamin A, iron, potassium, and calcium, just to name a few...

**Pound for pound, Moringa has:**

- 7 times the vitamin C found in oranges
- 4 times the calcium found in milk, and twice the protein
- 4 times the vitamin A found in carrots
- 3 times the potassium found in bananas
- 3 times the iron found in almonds

And, it's so much EASIER to take
a multivitamin, isn't it?

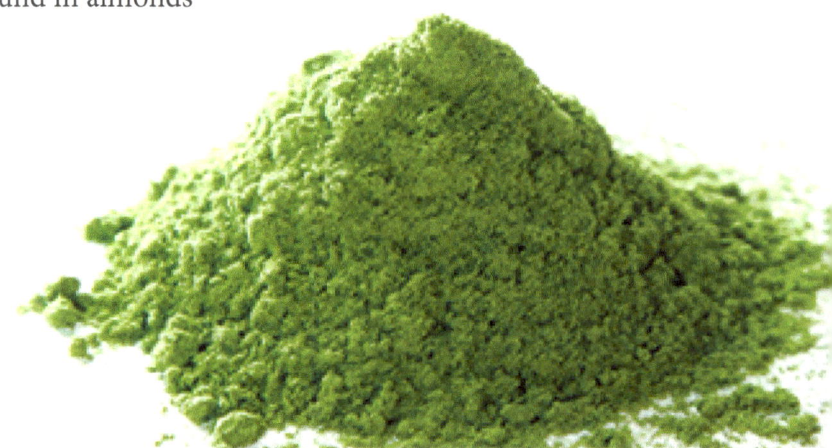

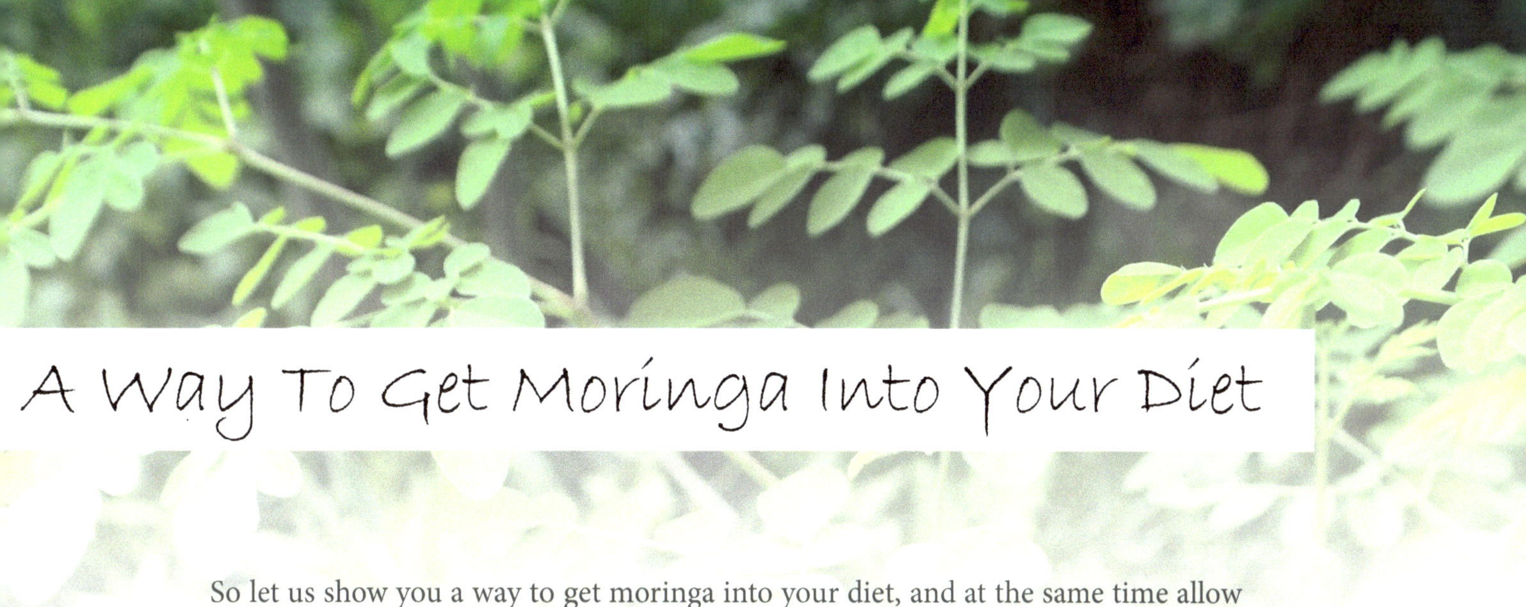


So let us show you a way to get moringa into your diet, and at the same time allow you to throw that next-to-useless multivitamin in the trash.

**What we are about to share with you has… an abundance of Moringa in its scientifically-proven dosage…**

Is guaranteed authentic, direct from the source…
Is 100% organic
Costs less than $1.36 per day
And is absolutely delicious…

It's so tasty in fact, we drink a tall glass of this each and every day.  And it tastes delicious!

**Plus Moringa is only one of ELEVEN nutrients in this elixir, each with their own fat-burning, anti-aging properties.**

**Find Out More In The Presentation Here  =>  http://bit.do/green-juice**

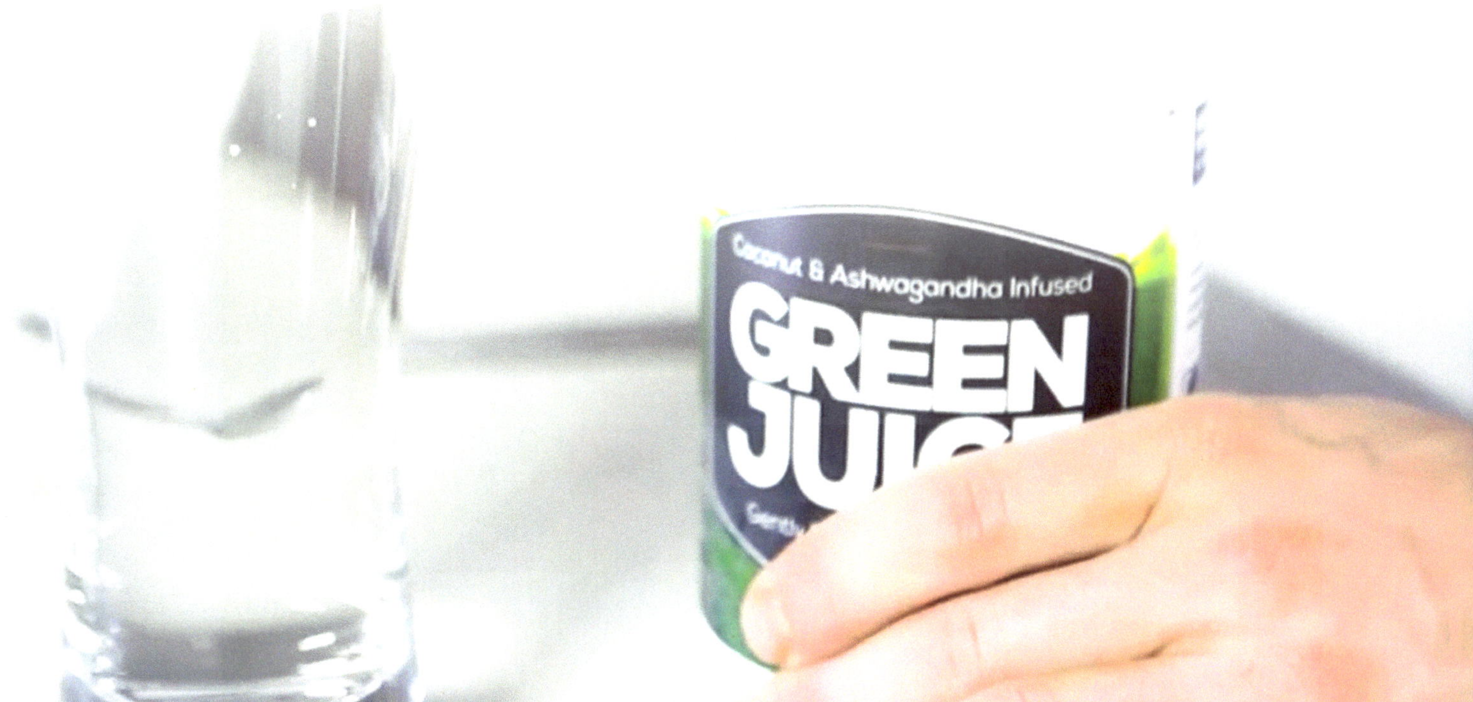

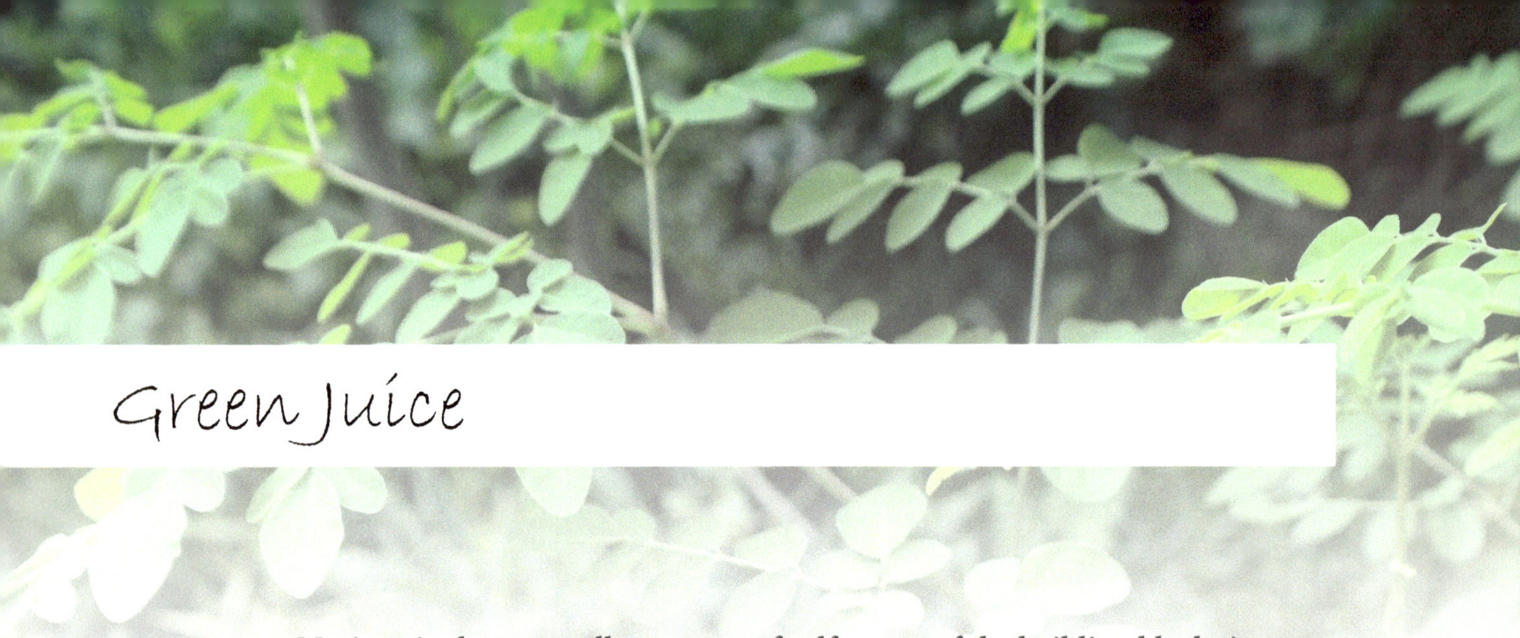

# Green Juice

Moringa is also an excellent source of sulfur, one of the building blocks in your collagen that <u>keeps skin tight and elastic.</u>

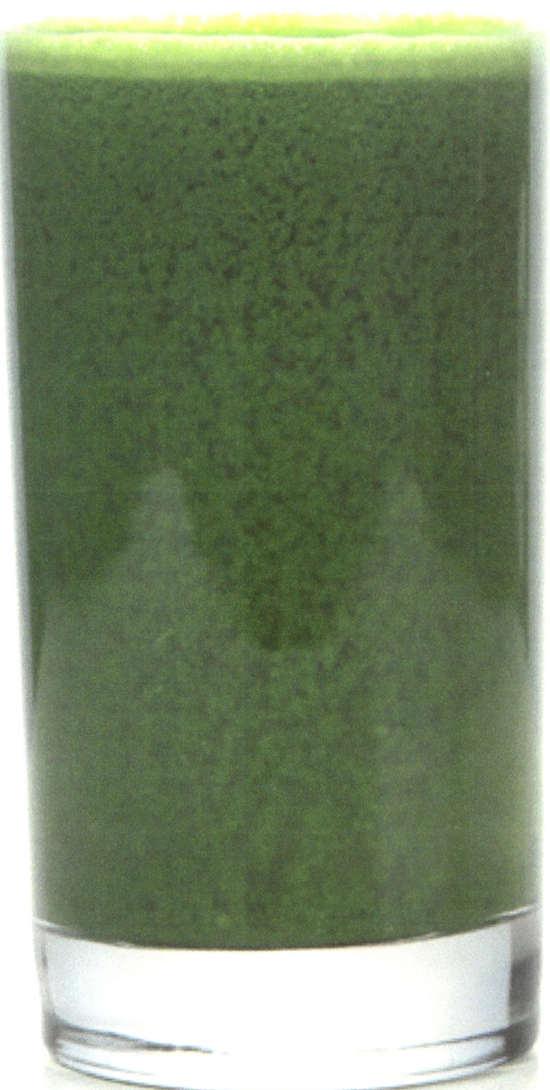

Plus the plethora of nutrients and antioxidants work to strengthen nails and keep hair thick and lustrous.

**>> So this delicious beverage helps you burn fat, strengthen the immune system, boost energy AND makes you look younger?**

Take a sip now while it's at a limited-time reduced price.

**Find Out More In The Presentation Here:**

[http://bit.do/green-juice](http://bit.do/green-juice)

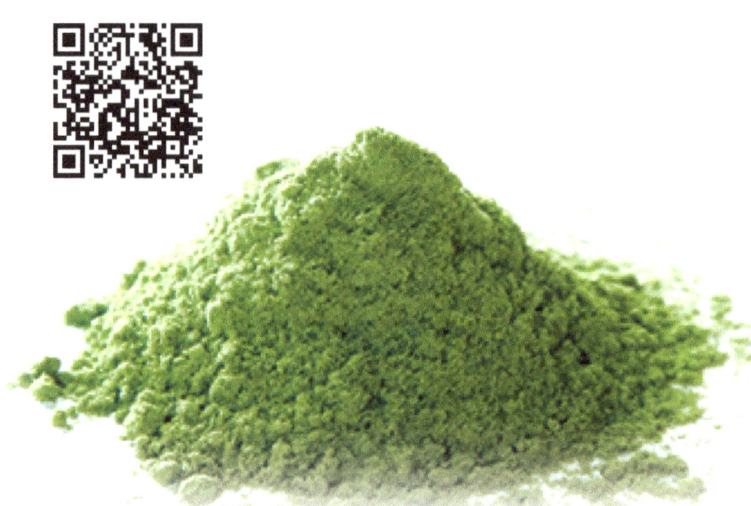